Making Sense
of Menopause

Making Sense
of Menopause

Harnessing the Power and
Potency of Your Wisdom Years

SUSAN WILLSON, CNM

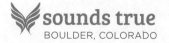
sounds true
BOULDER, COLORADO

Sounds True
Boulder, CO 80306

This book is not intended as a substitute for the medical recommendations
of physicians or other health-care providers. Rather, it is intended to offer
information to help the reader cooperate with physicians and health-care
providers in a mutual quest for optimum well-being. We advise readers to
carefully review and understand the ideas presented and to seek the advice of a
qualified professional before attempting to use them.

Published 2022

Cover design by Tara DeAngelis
Book design by Meredith March

Cover art by Tara DeAngelis

The wood used to produce this book is from
Forest Stewardship Council (FSC) certified forests,
recycled materials, or controlled wood.

Printed in the United States of America

BK06161

Library of Congress Cataloging-in-Publication Data

Names: Willson, Susan, author.
Title: Making sense of menopause : harnessing the power and potency of your
    wisdom years / Susan Willson, CNM.
Description: Boulder, CO : Sounds True, 2022.
Identifiers: LCCN 2021027409 (print) | LCCN 2021027410 (ebook) | ISBN
    9781683647447 (trade paperback) | ISBN 9781683647454 (ebook)
Subjects: LCSH: Middle-aged women–Psychology. | Menopause–Psychological
    aspects. | Self-actualization (Psychology) | Creative ability.
Classification: LCC BF724.6 .W56 2022 (print) | LCC
BF724.6 (ebook) | DDC 155.6/6–dc23
LC record available at https://lccn.loc.gov/2021027409
LC ebook record available at https://lccn.loc.gov/2021027410

10 9 8 7 6 5 4 3 2 1

For my daughter Gwen
who raised me right

We actually do come with Operating Instructions. They are coded in our DNA, in our conscience, in what draws our soul. It is not so important that we look successful in the world's eyes. What is important is that we live *our* life . . . the life we came here to live. We need to honor the incarnation we find ourselves in. No one else can live that life, give that gift. We must pay attention, listen . . . deeply . . . to ourselves, to what we move toward and to what brings us *joy*. Life is meant to be joyful, and if we can manage that, regardless of our circumstances, it transforms everything around us.   —**Susan Willson**

Contents

PART THREE Midlife Course Corrections

PART FOUR Moving Through

Introduction

Menopause

It's Not What You Think

There is something infinitely healing in the repeated
refrains of nature—the assurance that dawn comes after
night, and spring after the winter.   —Rachel Carson

There is a cultural belief in the West that menopause is an unavoidable horror. Prepare yourself, dig in, because this is going to be a wild ride. The hot flashes, sleep deprivation, fatigue, brain fog, hair loss, and the sense that everything is falling apart are seen on the horizon, headed for us, and we dread it. We feel helpless. These are the stories we hear and the way many women experience menopause, perhaps because it is what we are expecting. But why should this be so? Why would Nature create our bodies to suddenly unravel and leave us feeling lost and diminished, just when we are in the prime of our lives?

In a woman's biological story, the times of hormonal change are often a bit challenging to navigate. Things are shifting on a deeper level than just our bodies and we know this intuitively. We tend to think of ourselves as the same person throughout our life, someone that changes are happening *to*. But in a very real sense, our hormones literally change us into a different being at each juncture of our life as a woman. In the same way that a caterpillar and butterfly have exactly the same DNA but are very different creatures, we also go through a metamorphosis at times of hormonal change and do best if we embrace our new state of being rather than resisting or just trying to adapt. All of these times of change in our lives fit together and build, one upon the other. So, in order to navigate our menopause, we must also understand the earlier phases of our lives and how they connect to what is happening now, because they impact strongly what kind of menopause we will experience.

Unfortunately, menopausal women in Western culture are marginalized, made to feel "less than"; and make no mistake, cultural expectation is *very* powerful. For example, I once read about a primitive culture that held the belief that when women stopped menstruating they would die, so the women in that tribe menstruated well into their seventies. Their bodies complied. Whether or not the story is actually true, the principle is. In cultures where social status increases after menopause and there is no negative connotation to elderhood, women do not experience what we think of as menopausal symptoms to the same degree that Western women do, if at all. In other words, our bodies, minds, and beliefs are *one*.

In Western culture, the dominant message is that our bodies will betray us. In our profit-driven health-care system, disease is marketed to us in such a way that we see it waiting around every corner, and we often see the smallest symptoms in our bodies as harbingers of life-changing dysfunction. We buy this message because many of us are no longer in touch with what is true about our bodies.

We live in the midst of so much "noise chaos." We are asked to keep up with multiple times the tasks and amounts of information than we were even twenty years ago, and women in menopause today still remember older ways of being. We adapt, but we are aware of how much more we have to hold now. In today's world, we so rarely have the quiet, in our minds and bodies, to remember who we are. In this book, I invite you to stop for a minute, take a breath, and remember that Nature has a plan.

Nature—What Was She Thinking?

Nature provides each species with a blueprint for its unfolding, from the first moment of its existence. We watch birds, fish, and butterflies migrate across the globe with unerring accuracy to places they have never been. We watch flowers bud, blossom, and then wither in order to bear fruit. When we step back and watch from a distance, we can see that Nature's plan is elegant and systematic, but we don't trust it in the same way when it applies to our own bodies. We have been *taught* to fear death and aging.

Human physical, spiritual, and intellectual development also unfolds according to a plan, with each stage building upon the last, but from where we stand as individuals, we can only see where we are and have been. Having mentors and models who show us the way can help, but we are generally either past- or present-focused in terms of what we would say that we actually *know* or have mastered. Change is hard, and contemplating the future or the unknown, particularly in our current culture, carries an undercurrent of anxiety or fear for most people.

One aspect of Nature's unfolding program in humans is what we call aging. There are those who would say that, theoretically, we shouldn't *have* to age, that we have systems for regeneration in the body, if we just knew how to use them. (All cells in the body are made new on a constant basis, after all.) However, most of us are watching the lines form, the gray hair come in, and gravity take hold, and feeling a sense of inevitability about it. Some women feel despair.

When it comes to aging, not many of us are able to embrace and embody it. Most of us try to ignore it at best, come to fear it at worst, and that fear can put our bodies in survival mode, causing stress hormone levels to rise and putting forces into motion that actually quicken the physical signs of aging. To embrace and work with Nature's program as it unfolds is an option less taken but one that carries with it a sense of balance and rightness. I invite you to engage with this in a powerful way—to be open to the unknown and what you might find, to tell yourself the truth, and to receive the gifts this will certainly bring.

While Nature's plan for women is the same across the species, the journey we each make is a personal one. How we feel about being a woman in midlife (and beyond) is influenced by many things: our past experiences, the culture we live in and learn to define ourselves by, and the role models we have for aging, as well as the messages of our medical and religious communities that teach a separation between body and soul that doesn't serve us when we are working toward integration. In the West, we live in a culture that deifies youth and in which status is based on "looking good." What that means to each woman might differ, depending on the circle in which she travels. "Looking good" might be based on physical looks, the things she acquires, the power she wields, or her ease in different social situations.

As we will see in the following chapters, our individual stories as to how we experience menopause and aging actually begin in the womb. In fact, they begin in the three months prior to our conception. Understanding the path of our individual journey, and untangling ourselves from the various roles and identities we have inhabited in our lives up to this point, goes a long way toward bringing us to a place of authenticity and thriving during menopause and beyond. This in turn lessens symptoms and anxiety and provides us with a strong place to stand in the world.

So, while it might seem odd in a book about menopause to first read about how we come to be female and experience puberty and menstruation, it *is* relevant because our earliest experiences really do shape our menopause. This journey begins at the beginning.

The Journey

As a Nurse Midwife, I have cared for women through all phases of their lives. However, my practice for the last twenty years has been focused on working with women in the menopausal transition, and there is a common shape to the journey. When a woman first comes into my office, she is often feeling desperate. She is experiencing changes to her body, mood, sleep patterns, libido, and ability to focus. She is also vaguely aware that there is a deeper sea change happening, that something bigger than her symptoms is at work under the surface. A raw power is rising up, but it feels out of control and very different from what has come before. This adds to her anxiety. She may fear that her body is irretrievably broken. She is looking for answers, for relief, and at least for the moment, to be "fixed." She wants things to be the way they were, even if they weren't great, because at least they were familiar, something she knows she can cope with.

I remind her that her life as a woman is a continuum and one that is very much influenced by hormonal status. I suggest that she reflect on what her responses were during other times of major hormonal shift in her life. If she is like most women, there was likely a sense of being off-balance, not knowing who she was anymore, not knowing what this new role would ask of her or how to navigate it. Yet once the transition was made, she found her feet and moved forward to inhabit the next phase of her life. I remind her that Nature has a plan in place for us, as it does for all beings in the world, and we can look forward to it with curiosity and anticipation. I remind her, "You've got this. You have so much to draw on and everything you need to become the next best version of yourself."

Many of you reading this book might be in a similar place. You want to make sense of what is happening to you, you want to feel *normal* again, but you don't yet have a sense of what that new normal might be. It can be a very scary place to be, especially without cultural support. This book will help you.

Remember, Western medicine generally wants to isolate and "fix" our symptoms. It sees menopause as an inevitable failure of the fertility system. Yet menopause is not something to be "fixed" or even something that *can* be fixed. It is a natural process, not a syndrome, and an initiation—physical, emotional, and developmental—that each of us as women must go through. We bring to that process who we are, by way of our personal histories and methods of coping. Our histories and experiences shape not only *what* happens but also how we respond to it, how long it will last, and what the outcomes will be. Once women begin to really explore their journeys through childhood, girlhood, and womanhood, they generally find that their ways of being, their problems, whatever is yet "undone" in their lives become amplified and distilled during this time.

Menopause truly is a crossroads. Women will generally either embrace it and move through it thriving, or begin to slowly diminish. This is why our individual stories are so important, and why it is important for women to tell them, if they are going to heal whatever is undone in their lives and bring themselves whole into the next phase. We need to hear one another's stories, learn from them, and realize that we are not alone.

I always make sure that the women I work with have an opportunity to tell and explore their stories, and that they have someone to listen to them. Healing cannot occur without that. The old adage "Wherever you go, there you are" is never more true than when talking about menopause. How a woman frames the events of her life, what her expectations are, and how willing she is to be vulnerable and explore past patterns that no longer serve her have huge implications for her in terms of how she will experience menopause and navigate the rest of her life.

In addition, her lifestyle and stress levels will have a direct impact on symptoms. For one woman, minor lifestyle adjustments or a small dose of hormone to help her get back into balance is all she needs; she feels "herself" again. Another woman, with a different history, may need an extended period of working on adrenal health and some more serious lifestyle changes before she begins to feel more normal. For yet another, therapy or some other form of process work to complete unfinished business or resolve past trauma is what makes the difference. Sadly, some women address none of this, experience hot flashes and other symptoms into their seventies, and never truly feel well again. But it doesn't have to be that way.

How a woman feels about her female identity, what stories she has been told, the presence or absence of sexual trauma—all of these things will affect a woman's experience of menopause and the degree to which she experiences symptoms. So, following the breadcrumbs from our earliest life can highlight where symptoms originate from and allow us to better target the work that needs to be done to bring ourselves whole to the next part of our journey. The Going Deeper sections of this book are designed to help you do this.

The Fruits of the Journey

Midlife can be a time of deepening insight, increased confidence, freedom from reproductive concerns; a creative time when there is an intersection of wisdom and creativity that Nature supports; a time to give our gift to the world. In fact, anthropologists tell us that grandmothers furthered the evolution of our species. Once women survived long enough to be grandmothers, they gathered the most food. They also had the time and patience to teach children and the life experience to contemplate consciousness beyond survival, waking up a totally different part of the human brain.

One thing is certain: menopause is a critical juncture. It is a point at which women generally decide to move forward and embrace their elderhood and the wisdom they have accumulated or they begin to give up and fade away.

I have found that most women, once their symptoms are under better control and they have the emotional bandwidth again, *want* to do the work that will help them catch up to present time, to find out what is authentic for them *now* and how they want to express this going forward. They want to live vibrant lives into their elder years. This doesn't just happen, though. This, too, is a process that requires attention.

Sifting through how we became who we are and what the stories are that we have been living is a powerful, engaging, and profoundly moving process. It is *important* that we look back through our lives to honor and assess, grieve and celebrate the things we have been, done, and lost. We cannot fully become the "next thing" without that. However, ours is not a culture that knows how to grieve or that supports grieving, except in the most private of places. Too many women stay trapped in the loss and are unable to move on to the next phase—fully inhabiting themselves and opening to the incredible richness that midlife and elderhood can bring. We cannot do this work effectively while we are in the midst of a downward spiral. We first need to support ourselves back to balance.

This book gives you the tools and opportunity to do both—to understand what is happening in your body and to take some steps to rebalance it. Throughout the course of the book, we will explore the overall arc of a woman's biological life, where menopause fits into this, and how each of the passages we have already completed impacts our menopause. We will see how each of our former transitions relates to and informs what we are going through now and how Nature prepares us for each phase. We will explore what we can do to care for ourselves, lessen symptoms we might be having, and come back to a place of balance and equilibrium.

Perhaps even more important, we will begin to explore our stories, because our earliest experiences and the stories we have used to frame our identities largely inform what kind of menopause we will experience, not our genetics. Looking at our personal stories helps us remember who we have been, and from there to see who we are now, what is authentic to our truest selves at this juncture, and what is not. Knowing that and catching up to present time allows us to move into this next phase of our lives whole, knowing what we want from it and what we wish to give. Elderhood can be the most powerful phase of our lives, and as we will see going forward, allows us to shape our culture and those who come after us.

How to Use This Book

This book is structured so that you can use it in whatever way meets your needs best at this time. The story of each step along the biological path of a woman's life is presented first, and how it relates to where you are now. How Nature's plan unfolds to prepare us for each new phase is a fascinating story that may surprise you. These sections will help you understand what is happening in your body and provide ways that you can work with what is happening to create vibrant health for yourself, wherever you are along that path.

Working with the Going Deeper sections at the end of each chapter will help you understand your personal journey, where you have come from, and what people and experiences have been most potent in shaping the way you think of yourself and the way you present in the world. These sections take you a little deeper into some of the issues we have discussed in each chapter and how they relate to your life.

Being aware of your own trajectory will help to increase your understanding of where you currently stand in terms of your health and the issues you face. Seeing the path that brought you to where you are now will help you make the adjustments that will ensure vibrancy in your future. It can also help you to be more compassionate and accepting of your current situation, which is invaluable when trying to make change.

Some of these questions may attract you; some may hold no draw at all. There is no right way to approach them. You might decide to start a journal in which to write down what information you find and your responses to it. If you are comfortable, talk with your mother or other family members about the questions pertaining to your early life. See what information they can provide and what their experiences were. Then see what floats to the surface. If you have a trusted friend or therapist, you might choose to talk about what feelings arise in you based on what you find out. You might have a group of women with whom you wish to explore this journey, and there are a wealth of benefits to doing this work in a group. Hearing the stories of others and receiving accurate mirroring helps bring perspective and compassion.

I have clients who work with this information by just thinking about it, and those who decide to write or make art that reflects their journey. For some, an "aha" moment that comes from something they find out completely changes the way they understand an experience or some old pattern they are held by. Whatever you choose to do with it, this knowledge creates a framework and context that you can use to look at your current state of being, and from there you can move forward. I would encourage you to move toward what speaks to you and set aside some contemplative time for this process.

There is no rush, and this inquiry yields the best results if you engage with it slowly and only engage when you have the emotional energy to do so. Many women will want to just read through the book once and let things percolate, get used to the ideas presented here, then go back to whatever section seems to call to them, when they are ready. This journey will have a timing all its own.

Thoughts at the end of each Going Deeper section will help you take what you have learned and consolidate the gold there so that it can be useful to you. Throughout the course of the book, you can chart your own journey from girlhood to maidenhood to midlife and create a path for the future that draws you forward with curiosity and excitement, to live fully and give the gift of your life's learning to the world.

Women who are in the thick of symptoms may wish to skip to the chapter on self-care. If you do so, I encourage you to then go back and begin at the beginning. For example, knowing your origins and how your brain is wired in regard to stress can help you better understand your current stress levels in a way that allows you to address them more effectively and thereby decrease many of your menopausal symptoms.

For those who have the curiosity and the emotional energy available right now, I strongly encourage you to explore the book in order, from beginning to end, taking time with the self-inquiry and building up to present time. While this is deeply personal work, it can be even richer if engaged in with trusted others, who can help you reflect and find the gold in this investigation. So, I would encourage you to draw together a circle of companions specific to this journey and create a space just for this, so that you can give it your full focus and attention, outside of life's many distractions.

Even if you are not yet in menopause, this book and the journey it will take you on can still be very useful to you if you want to know more about yourself and your body. It will help those in the premenopausal years to prepare for the transition that's coming, making it possible to move through it with fewer symptoms and more grace and ease. We always feel safer if we are confident and prepared. This book is written out of a profound respect for women, the human spirit, and what women at this time of life, when our culture wants to diminish us, have to give.

I honor and respect that self-identity in regard to gender is a fluid thing, and that those of us in female bodies fall along that spectrum and use different pronouns to identify ourselves. But all of us, unless we have made a hormonal transition, will experience menopause. When discussing hormones and their effect on the body, and Nature's plan for reproduction, there will be a heterosexual focus, as reproduction requires male and female biology. I hope, however, that everyone will feel welcome here and find the book useful. I have used the word *partner* in most places in this book, rather than assuming any gender for one's partner (except where it is clear we are talking about a man), and I have used the pronoun *she* in order to simplify the writing. But know that you are included here, whatever pronouns you use to identify yourself. Names of any clients mentioned have been changed to protect their privacy.

Because we are often overwhelmed with the many demands of our multitasking lives, it can seem impossible to know where to begin to find the place in ourselves that is true and *authentic* in the world. Far from being a time of endings and loss, as our culture frames it, menopause is a time of becoming, and I find it infinitely reassuring that Nature has programming already in place for us. This is part of the Plan. It is just a matter of falling back into a deep pool, listening, unfolding into, and finally nourishing ourselves in the ways that we have nourished others for so long. When we do, the gifts of menopause are profound.

PART ONE

It Begins at
the Beginning

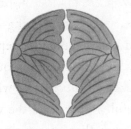

Chapter 1

The Continuum

All our knowledge has its origins in our
perceptions.   —Leonardo da Vinci

A college professor of mine once said, "You can pull any thread and unravel the Universe." At nineteen, that opened up for me an image of the interconnectedness of the Universe that was more fluid than the one I was working with at the time, which looked something like puzzle pieces. That statement is never more true than when looking at how the many different processes in our bodies relate to one another, particularly hormone balance.

How we tend to think of ourselves in terms of our hormones is generally frozen at a certain point on the time line of our lives. We might say we are "latent" at ten years old, in the "prime of our reproductive years" in our twenties and thirties, "winding down" into our late forties, or menopausal in our sixties. In truth, rather than being a series of distinct phases, our hormonal life is a long and very fluid continuum. Where we find ourselves hormonally at any given point in time is informed by things that happened years ago, as far back as the hormonal balance of our mothers before we were even conceived.

We begin as fairly androgynous beings. At the time of puberty, we experience a hormonal surge (estrogen for women, testosterone for men), which polarizes us for purposes of reproduction and literally turns us into different creatures, in the same way that a caterpillar is quite distinct from a butterfly in its appearance, characteristics, and longings, even as one has its beginnings in the other and they share exactly the same DNA. These changes are not just in the realm of our physiognomy but encompass every aspect of our being—how the brain works and what areas are being stimulated, how cells function, what our emotional state is, what drives behavior, and how we respond to the world around us.

We quite literally go through a metamorphosis when we go through our hormonal changes. Just as a caterpillar and butterfly are expressions of the same creature yet different in form, function, makeup, and destiny, so our hormones change us into different creatures as we move from girlhood through puberty and our reproductive years and into our Wisdom years. While not every woman experiences pregnancy and the tidal wave of hormonal change that brings, those who do don't miss for a second the fact that they are a very different creature when pregnant and that those changes are something over which they have no control. The same is true at each hormonal shift.

These times of metamorphosis are critical junctures in the unfolding of the human biological program and the evolving of our consciousness. Our bodies, our patterns, our possibilities all open up at these times when things are made new. We are given the opportunity to re-form in a different pattern, as well as complete any unfinished business from the stage preceding. For instance, we have hormonal support during pregnancy to make the changes necessary to our brain and body to create a new human being, begin mothering, and nurse a baby. Likewise, hot flashes herald the transition to the Wisdom years, when hormones stimulate creative centers in the brain that entice us into the next phase of life, where our creative endeavors are given priority.

Our hormones mediate every aspect of our biology. They are the cellular messengers that make it possible for us to adapt moment to moment and over time to our environment. While we are most familiar with the sex hormones estrogen and testosterone, hormones are fundamental to all the systems of the body. They regulate our growth, metabolism, stress levels, blood pressure, and blood sugar. They are the chemical messengers the body uses to communicate with itself in the constant process of call and response that regulates its systems. We will talk about some of these in detail in later chapters of the book.

Hormones powerfully change us from girls into women capable of reproducing, into mothers capable of giving birth and nursing an infant, into elders capable of evolving our species. Our ancestral grandmothers strengthened our tribes. They ensured the survival of older children, thereby making it possible for mothers to have more children who survived. They were the memory keepers and held the time line of our history.

We Are Made to Adapt

Our bodies are exquisite adaptation machines. We know that the human body has not changed very much since we arrived on the planet. That being so, Nature must have a way to prepare each baby for the world it is being born into. This process begins in the three months before ovulation of the egg that will become you.

When scientists unraveled the human genome (the complete set of genes for the human body), they found far fewer genes than they were expecting. The prevailing view at the time was that genes were causative—each gene was responsible for creating a specific trait or disease. What they found instead was that genes are either turned on or turned off based on what the environment tells them is needed. As it turns out, the prime directive of the human body is to adapt.

Cell biologist Bruce Lipton, who did much of the early research on gene expression at Stanford University in the mid-1980s, can take you step by step through the process that shows that our health and our gene expression are mediated on a cellular level by our *perceptions* of our environment—not just what our environment was or is but our *perception* of that environment. (See *The Biology of Belief: Unleashing the Power of Consciousness, Meaning and Miracles,* by Bruce Lipton.) In fact, a whole new branch of science has developed in the last two decades exploring this, called *epigenetics* (meaning "above genetics"). Beliefs are powerful.

So, a gene will express or not, depending on what messages it receives from the environment and what beliefs we hold about the environment we inhabit. Our personal stories begin here. Let's look at how this thread, this continuum, might run through a life.

Three months before ovulation, gene sequencing begins in the egg based on the environmental signals that come through the hormones of the mother's body. Remember, hormones are the chemical messengers that tell the body what is required moment to moment. If your mother's life was moderately stressful in the months leading up to your birth, this could affect your hormonal balance even now, at age fifty-five, as you move through menopause.

It happens like this: Stress hormones in your mother's body inform the gene sequencing in the developing egg, as to what traits will be needed to be best suited for the environment it will potentially be born into. The egg most suited to the environment at the time of ovulation launches. Once you are conceived, as your fetal brain develops, the level of your mother's stress hormones will continue to inform brain development, strengthening the pathways that sensitize stress response if the mother's life is very stressful, or using that energy for development in different areas if it is not.

Nature wants to prepare each baby for the world it is being born into, so a baby born into a war-torn country would need to have a more sensitive stress response, if it is to survive, than a baby born into a sleepy town in the Midwest. Or at least this is the way Mother Nature sees it. So, if a pregnant woman is experiencing constant stress, those stress hormones tell the developing fetal brain that the world is a dangerous place and it had better be prepared. That baby, when it is born, will be more likely to go into stress response more quickly and fully in the presence of environmental stressors than one whose mother had a tranquil pregnancy. The baby is literally "wired" to do so. Further life experiences will strengthen this response.

This sensitivity to stress comes into play during perimenopause and menopause, strongly influencing our hormone levels and hormone balance, and therefore our symptoms. Nature will *always* prioritize survival over reproduction. In fact, Nature does not want you to be pregnant if you are under a great deal of stress, because pregnancy is a state of high energy use. So, when there is stress, everything tilts toward making stress hormones and not the sex hormones needed for reproduction. Lower levels of these sex hormones, in the presence of stress, will cause more symptoms of perimenopause and menopause.

All sex hormones (estrogen, progesterone, testosterone) and stress hormones (cortisol, adrenaline, DHEA, norepinephrine) are made from the same raw material. They are all based on the cholesterol molecule, and Nature has made it so that, with very few exceptions, hormones can change into one another depending on what is needed in the body at any given moment, with the addition of some simple chemical subgroups, such as oxygen. This capacity is part of what makes the body so adaptable.

So, if there is stress, the body's first priority is to make stress hormones to aid survival, and it makes fewer sex hormones (even if the body is low in them and "needs" them). Fast-forward to when the baby, who was wired for stress, is now a woman. Her body goes into stress response more easily. If the adrenal glands, which make the stress hormones, are overtired and cannot make enough, her body will literally steal the sex hormones and turn them into stress hormones, making her "deficient" in progesterone, testosterone, and, if unchecked, estrogen and thereby cause symptoms of hormone deficiency. This will translate into more premenstrual syndrome (PMS) when she is in her reproductive years, or more hot flashes and other symptoms when she is in her menopausal years.

We Are Made to Survive

To continue with our story, the baby with the more sensitive stress response will go into fight-or-flight more easily throughout her life than her counterpart who experienced a tranquil pregnancy. The fight-or-flight response, initiated by the adrenal glands, is the body's response to stress that ensures our survival.

Our adrenal glands, two tiny pyramid-shaped glands that sit on top of our kidneys, are what mediate stress in our bodies. Day to day, they help to provide energy for moment-to-moment activities, regulate blood pressure and blood sugar, and decrease inflammation. They are also involved in our immune response.

According to our original design, if we ran into a mastodon on the plain, the adrenals would produce a tidal wave of hormones, putting us into an altered state for two to three hours so that we could run faster, fight harder, or climb a higher tree, thereby helping us to survive the encounter. If we escaped the mastodon, our hormone levels would return to normal after a couple of hours and stay there until our next emergency, which likely was not fifteen minutes later.

The way we live today is quite different. However, the brain doesn't really distinguish much between running into a mastodon on the plain and being stuck in traffic, overwhelmed with work, fighting with our spouse, struggling through a long physical illness, or having to be available 24/7 by phone, email, or messaging.

To the brain, stress is stress. So, it is literally possible for a modern person to be in a fight-or-flight response almost twenty-four hours a day, because the stress response lasts an average of two to three hours and can be triggered over and over during the day. For the woman wired for stress as a baby, this is often the case.

It is even possible for the fight-or-flight response to be triggered while we are sleeping at night, due to a drop in blood sugar. The brain is safe only within a very narrow range of blood sugar, and the body wants to keep the brain safe at all costs, since it is running the show. Therefore, we have a very delicate mechanism in place to regulate blood sugar.

When our blood sugar gets too high, the hormone insulin rises and stores that sugar as fat. On the other hand, when our blood sugar drops too low and there is no food coming in, fight-or-flight is activated in the body and our liver empties its emergency stores of sugar and fat into the bloodstream to give us quick energy. This is the first step in the fight-or-flight process. The rush of adrenaline that accompanies this is what wakes up many menopausal women at 2:30 or 3:30 a.m. out of a sound sleep and then makes them unable to get back to sleep for two hours (the amount of time the fight-or-flight response lasts). So, keeping blood sugar stable is a very good strategy to improve sleep during menopause.

Early woman had a benefit that we don't have. If she survived the mastodon, the stress hormones in her body would be cleared from her bloodstream by running, fighting, or climbing that tree. We do not usually get that opportunity. Our stress hormones, rather than being used for fighting or fleeing and then metabolized out of the body, hang around in tissues and metabolize more slowly. We modern women stay in a constant state of "stew and chew" rather than moving through fight-or-flight as Nature intended.

A woman who is sensitized to stress by high levels of stress hormones as a developing baby, or as a young child, will tend to perceive her environment as stressful when another might not. This pattern will continue to reinforce itself over her lifetime, and she will likely arrive at menopause with very tired adrenal glands.

As part of Nature's plan, the adrenal glands and fat cells are supposed to take over hormone production for the second half of life, when the ovaries wind down. (During this time, many women develop what is jokingly called the "meno-pot," an extra five pounds of fat padding their waistlines, which is needed for making hormones and which the body is very happy to provide!) If the adrenals are already tired at the time they are asked to take on this extra job, as well as being expected to keep up with day-to-day stress needs, they often go into a tailspin. They simply cannot do it all, and the body spirals downward in the presence of low levels of hormones, causing symptoms to occur.

I have had many a woman say to me, "I don't know *what* happened. Yes, life is stressful, but it is no worse than usual. I am handling it. It is nothing I haven't done before. Then I started missing a few periods and suddenly I have hot flashes and night sweats. I am irritable, exhausted, my hair is falling out, my knees hurt, I can't sleep at night, and I am hungry all the time. I am gaining weight like crazy! WHAT is going on? How can just missing a couple of periods cause all this?" These women feel very afraid because everything seems out of control.

I explain to them that it is not just the fact that they missed a couple of periods but that they have likely arrived at this juncture in their lives with very tired adrenals and there is nothing left to take over, as the ovaries wind down their production of estrogen. Things can begin to spiral downward quickly in this situation as the body tilts all hormone production toward survival.

It Is All Connected

This is but one possible story of how our preconception life can affect our menopausal symptoms. There are many. Remember, "you can pull any thread and unravel the universe." Everything is connected to everything else in the body. The hormonal dance is an intricate game of Marco Polo, or echolocation, with a message being sent out and then an answering "ping." The answering message determines the next signal, because the body wants to be up to date at all times.

It can be easy to feel overwhelmed when we realize how interconnected everything is, but the message truly is a positive one. It means you *always* have the opportunity and the capability to come back into balance. Change the "Marco!" and the answering "Polo" will be different as well. As we have established, we are organisms exquisitely made for adaptation. The human body aims not only to survive but also to thrive in whatever environment it finds itself. This means we have the power of Nature supporting us as we try to make changes in our lives.

Going Deeper

The Shape of Our Journey

Being aware of your own life's trajectory can increase understanding of where you find yourself now, in terms of your health and the issues you might face during your menopausal years. Knowing your story will help you begin to see the path you have been on thus far and highlight adjustments that will help to ensure vibrant health for your future. It will also allow you to be more compassionate and accepting of where you are now, which is invaluable when trying to make change—especially as you move through menopause and into your elder years.

Since this is very early information, check with family members if you need to in order to find answers. Consider the following questions:

- What do you know about your mother's life just before she became pregnant with you? Were things particularly stressful emotionally, financially, socially? If so, why?

- Were there any deaths in the family while you were in the womb? If so, how did this affect the family you were being born into, your mother in particular?

- Is there any history in your family, especially your mother, of depression or any other mental health challenges that might affect stress levels or brain chemistry? If so, what?

- What was your mother's physical health like at the time she became pregnant with you? Did she smoke or use alcohol or drugs? Did she restrict calories? Were there complications to the pregnancy?

- What do you know about your birth? Were there complications? Was it a very long labor? Were you born vaginally or by cesarean section? Was there any instrumentation (forceps or vacuum extractor) used in your birth?

- Were you separated from your mother for physical reasons or hospital protocol, or were you able to stay with her right after birth? How might this have affected you or established an early pattern?

- Were you breastfed or bottle fed? How did your body respond to this food? Were you a colicky baby?

- Did you cry a lot? Were you hard to soothe? How might this have affected your mother's response to you?

- Were your parents happy with your gender or were they wishing for a child of the opposite sex? How was your femaleness received? What stories have you been told in this regard?

- What stories have you been told about your role in your birth (e.g., "You were in such a hurry, you just tore me apart . . . you couldn't wait," or "You just cried all the time; we thought there was something wrong with you").

- At what age were you given into the care of others (daycare, babysitters) so that your parents could work, or did you stay at home with a parent?

- What was the feeling tone of your early childhood? Do you remember it as happy? Safe? Stressful? Loving? What are some of the memories that inform this?

- Was your home in your early years a tranquil place, with enough food, parental love, and a sense of safety? Or was there fighting, financial issues, or other early stressors present in your home? If there was stress, were you aware of the cause or did you feel it had somehow to do with you?

- What is your first memory?

Answers to these questions will give you some insight into the stressors of your early life and what kind of place you thought the world to be when you were very young. It may surprise you to know that such early experiences can have a material effect on your menopause. These early impressions can be very potent in terms of setting lifelong sensitivities as to how you will be received, stress, and habits of view because the brain essentially acts like a tape recorder until about age six. It functions mostly in theta-wave state (very similar to a hypnotic state) and just "downloads" experience without the analytical capacity to make judgments about it.

You might wish to validate some of what you found in your self-inquiry with your mother or other family members. Gathering information from your womb time and infancy can be challenging, especially if your parents are no longer alive. If they are, mine these resources. It could increase your connection to family members, and the stories it elicits can be very illuminating. If your memories don't agree, what were their perspectives?

If you are unable to speak with a parent or someone who would have this early information but you want to explore it, hypnosis has been shown to be very effective at recovering early memories and sensations, even as far back as the womb. Also, since our very early memories effectively live in every cell of our bodies, you might wish to try one of the treatment modalities that can bypass your brain's analytic function and speak directly to your body. These include Somatic Experiencing, Craniosacral work, Brainspotting, Neurofeedback, Emotional Freedom Technique (tapping), Process Acupressure, and various forms of breathwork. These modalities can help to uncover early material and heal the body from the effects of trauma.

If you find that stress has been a long-term pattern in your life and you would like to address this, consider some proven ways to deal with stress such as meditation, massage, hypnotherapy, and exercise. Reconnecting with our earliest consciousness often helps us to remember our wholeness and why we are here.

Chapter 2

What Does It Mean
to Be Male or Female?

> I don't know if I know what being female means
> exactly, but when I figure it out I'll text you and
> let you know. —Grace, thirteen years old

This is really getting down to basics. How does being male or female relate to where you are now in menopause? *Simple*, you might say. *If I wasn't female, I wouldn't be going through this!* In fact, men go through it, too. It just looks a bit different.

However, the more important point is that being either male or female is not as cut and dried as we like to think it is. It is, again, a continuum. Where we fall on that continuum—how our brain unfolds, how our body receives and uses estrogen (what we think of as the "female" hormone), and how we come to think of ourselves as women—has a lot to do with how we will experience our menopause.

We generally think of the sex hormones coming into play at puberty, when girls and boys experience the surge of estrogen, progesterone, testosterone, and adrenal hormones that initiate the development of the physical sexual characteristics we associate with each gender. However, these hormones have their most profound impact on an individual in utero, around the eighth week of pregnancy, when they signal the developing fetus to become physically male or female—just having an X or Y chromosome is no guarantee. For a boy to be made, several things have to happen on time and in sequence; otherwise, the baby will express as female, regardless of the Y chromosome it carries.

In the eighth week of pregnancy, a gene on the Y (male) chromosome begins the development of male genitals. If this gene does not kick in and the testes do not develop and start making testosterone, male genitals will not develop. Even if male genitals begin to develop, they must also make a special hormone (called Müllerian inhibiting factor) that causes the fetal structures that would otherwise turn into a uterus and ovaries to atrophy or wither away. Even if both of these things happen as they should, a third piece of the process also needs to happen for a boy to be made: the tissue receptors on the structures that will become the penis need to be able to suck up testosterone and use it.

Here again, Nature's desire to cooperate shows itself. The Y chromosome needs the X chromosome to create proper male genitals. The X chromosome contains an androgen receptor gene that ensures that the tissues of developing male organs will be able to take up and use testosterone. If that gene is not functioning, then the male genitalia will not fully develop and outer labia will remain as separate lips and not fuse together to make a sac to hold the testicles. The tissue that has the potential to develop as either a clitoris or a penis will not enlarge to become a penis.

These babies, while genetically "male," will not only look female but will often grow up to look like our cultural ideal of the most luscious female—creamy skin, scant body hair, a lush crop of head hair—because they don't have receptors for testosterone. They will not be fertile, as their budding uteri and ovaries disappeared on cue, and they will generally have shortened vaginas, even though their (hidden) testicles continue to make testosterone. In most cases, these testicles are removed at full growth, and the young women are put on hormone replacement therapy for their estrogen. These XY women will also not go through menopause in the same way that XX women do, since they don't have ovaries. Their estrogen levels will diminish as they age, but generally not enough to cause symptoms.

So, a developing fetus can have the chromosomes that define it as male (XY), but if the hormonal dance does not unfold as Nature intended and testicular development is not initiated, the uterus and ovaries are not withdrawn, and the receptors for testosterone are not active, they will be born appearing female.

Children who develop testicles but do not produce the hormone to atrophy the female genitalia will end up with both ovarian and testicular tissue and be intersex (what used to be called hermaphrodite, having both male and female genitalia). Nature is nothing if not creative.

It used to be that when a baby was born intersex, the doctor (sometimes with parental input) would just decide what sex the child would "be" and body parts were removed or adjusted to better "fit" that gender. The belief was that the child would identify with whatever sex the baby was raised as. There has been a world of pain for many individuals wrapped up in that belief.

Thankfully, medical science and psychology are catching up, and these children are treated much more sensitively now than they used to be. Decisions are less arbitrarily made as to whether they will be raised male or female, and many families opt to "wait and see" and let their growing children discern their gender identity.

We have become increasingly aware in the last decade that gender identity is fluid and often has little to nothing to do with a person's external genitals at birth. Evidence shows that the level of hormone disruptors in the environment these days also has an effect on gender expression in humans and other species on the planet. While there is evidence that gender fluidity has been present as long as there have been humans, it is either expressing itself more often now or our current culture is more open to that expression.

It is, in fact, not accurate even to label a hormone as male or female, since both genders make and use all of the different sex hormones, just in different ratios. As we have seen, Nature is flexible, cooperative, and above all, adaptable.

As we grow, these hormones continue to surge and withdraw, informing brain, muscle, and bone, until puberty is reached and they begin to enact their most visible dance, which for girls is the budding of soft, curvy breasts and hips and the lengthening of swanlike necks and legs. You can see when the hormones "hit the brain." Even before they know what all of this is for, girls get a nice little swing to their hips, begin having more face time with their mirrors, and start to mimic their female role models. I still remember the day the red nail polish made its way onto my daughter's altar at age eleven, to sit among all of the rocks, crystals, and fairy statues—a portent of things to come.

Going Deeper

Our Early Gender Experiences

For women of our generation, issues of gender identity might not be quite so fluid as they are in the younger generation today. While you may not have questioned your gender identity, you were definitely targeted as a woman by advertising and pressured to think that femininity, or being a woman, was meant to look a certain way.

- How did you feel about being a girl?

- What were you told about yourself in terms of your worth as a girl, your feminine qualities?

- What were the downsides, if any, to being feminine in your world; were there restrictions placed on you? If so, what were they? Whose point of view was this?

- Were there things you wanted to do that you felt you couldn't pursue because of your gender?

- Did you feel feminine? Or did narrow cultural views of femininity make you feel that you were lacking somehow?

- Did you feel masculine? Were you able to integrate all the pieces of yourself growing up or were there some that needed to be put away in the context in which you lived?

- Prior to puberty, were you a tomboy? If so, at what age did this start to change, if it did? Was this from outside pressure or from within yourself?

- Did you enjoy living in your body when you were young? If so, did this change at puberty?

- Could you dress the way you wanted to? Express yourself the way you wanted to? Engage in the activities you wanted to pursue?

Our gender identity and the way we wish to express it sometimes shifts along a continuum during our lives. At midlife, many women discover that they no longer find value in fitting into cultural roles and expectations that restrict their self-expression.

If you are unable to comfortably express yourself in a way that truly reflects who you are in terms of gender, think about what it might take to do this. What is holding you back? Not being sure yourself? Family? The judgment of others?

For some women, coming closer to their authentic self-expression is something as simple as changing the way they dress or who they might choose to be intimate with. It might involve beginning an activity or learning something that you have always had an interest in but were told was not appropriate. If you have deeper feelings of discomfort, there is a wealth of information online and support for people who are more fluid along the gender spectrum. Most therapists have also been trained to support this exploration.

For many women, menopause is a time when they decide to fully express themselves and stop trying to fit into a mold someone else has created for them. It is a wonderful time to explore.

Chapter 3

Your Menstrual Cycle

At her first bleeding, a woman meets her power. During her bleeding years, she practices it. At menopause, she becomes it.   —**Traditional Native American saying**

With the onset of puberty comes the primal rhythm of the menstrual cycle. As women, we have all experienced a very intimate relationship with our monthly cycles, or the lack of them. We know the process engages all of us—our bodies, our brains, and our emotions. We feel the tidal pull toward that bright splash of blood each month in a way that is deep in our cells.

With the approach of menopause, this monthly drumbeat that marks our time begins to wane and then disappear. For many women, this feels like a huge loss, regardless of whether there are other symptoms. Other women are delighted. Whatever our relationship to our period, many of us do not fully understand what is happening each month and how it fits into other intertwined threads of our internal physical universe.

We have been taught in a very simplistic way about the menstrual cycle. Who of us does not remember the elementary and middle school "health" classes designed to teach us about what was happening in our bodies without ever mentioning our sexuality? In my day, we were shown animated films (brought to you by Kotex and Disney) and anatomical diagrams of the pelvis cut in half that looked nothing like what we were seeing between our legs. For many of us, our mothers were not likely to share much information, because they didn't have a lot to share. Their information was often scanty and their own sexuality largely hidden behind closed doors, even if they were experiencing it fully, because it was not considered proper to talk about it in public.

My mother tried. She did her best. She gave me the facts (which I had a hard time believing, given that I had essentially been brought up to believe that I didn't exist from the neck down), took me to a lecture given by the local pediatrician, and then handed me a book called *The Stork Didn't Bring You*. I remember reading chapter 11 on masturbation three times and still having no clue what they were talking about, because the language was so vague and the concept so far from anything I had been led to believe anyone would or should ever think about doing.

Whatever our initiation into these women's mysteries, most of us have grown up with the simple story that every month an egg follicle develops, is released, and either meets a sperm and becomes a baby or doesn't and results in a period. Actually, Nature is much more interesting than that. Nature is luscious. She's abundant. She wants us to have *many* opportunities to become pregnant. We don't produce two hundred to four hundred eggs at a time like salamanders and frogs, but we do have lots of backup.

Every month during her reproductive years, a woman's body develops up to twenty egg follicles (and I would suggest that *how* many has a lot to do with her current environment and stress levels). One of them becomes the primary follicle—the one the body considers most suited to the current conditions in its gene sequencing and potential (or two in the case of fraternal twins). This follicle is released, and its launching signals the brain to tell the others to stop developing. The remaining follicles then become hormone-producing cysts that help the one that made it on its journey. They produce the hormone progesterone to support the second half of the menstrual cycle. Progesterone is the "pro-gestational" hormone, the one that will support a pregnancy if there is a union of sperm and egg, until the placenta is developed enough to take over that job.

Progesterone has two primary jobs. One is to oppose the action of estrogen (which builds up the uterine lining). The other is to organize that uterine lining into the kind of spongy environment that will accept and nourish a fertilized egg if pregnant, or if not pregnant, that will slough off cleanly as a period, without leaving behind a lot of broken blood vessels.

Remember, though, that the brain and the rest of the body are playing Marco Polo. As long as the process is unfolding as intended, the correct signals will receive the correct corresponding responses and periods will be regular. However, if stress is particularly high, or the environment is full of hormone disruptors (certain plastics, pesticides, and many ingredients in cosmetics that bind to hormone receptors and act like hormones in the body), the signal coming back to the brain may not correspond well to the one that went out, and a hormone imbalance will occur.

For instance, many women, because of excess stress in their lives, do not develop as many egg follicles during their cycle, and what progesterone they do produce is sucked up by the adrenal glands and turned into cortisol (the main stress hormone) to handle stress requirements. Therefore, they don't have enough progesterone to do an adequate job of managing the uterine lining in the second half of their menstrual cycle. Without enough progesterone, the lining will keep growing and periods will be heavy or there will be bleeding in the middle of the cycle. This low progesterone level also creates the symptoms we think of as PMS—bloating, cramping, tender breasts, moodiness, difficulty sleeping, and food cravings—and will also make for a more difficult menopausal transition when the time comes.

Our perceptions can also affect how we experience our periods. Growing up, I was happy to have my period, as I was the last among my friends to start menstruating and I felt left out. I had cramps, sometimes bad ones, but had always seen my periods as healthy and the cramps as a natural part of that. I remember being totally thrown when my college roommate, who also had cramps, spoke of them saying, "I can just feel everything rotting in there." She routinely had horrible periods, and she saw her cramps as a distinctly unhealthy side effect. Chicken or egg? It is uncertain, but our *perception* of our environment, our reality, can create real physical symptoms.

I often felt lucky as a woman to have had that monthly opportunity to look at what was not being addressed in my life. The premenstrual time, when our buffer zone is thin, shows us very clearly what is not working in our lives, what we are not dealing with. If we are listening and honor what we hear, we will take a little extra downtime during our periods to nourish our bodies and reflect on our lives and what changes we need to make. This cyclic reminder to look at what is real for us can be an invaluable tool.

Becoming a Woman

How we were responded to as budding adolescents and initiated as women through our first periods heavily influences the development of our self-concept and self-esteem as women. Since the introduction of health and hygiene classes in public schools, most girls are somewhat prepared for menstruation these days. That was not always the case. Many girls in my generation started their first period and thought they were dying, because they found blood on their underwear one day and no one had told them to expect to bleed.

However, many girls who are prepared for this event are also steeped in attitudes of shame. They feel that menstruation should not be discussed and that somehow they are "unclean" while bleeding. Some religious proscriptions further this belief. Menstruation is an open secret in our current Western culture; most everyone is aware of the mechanics of menstruation, but most also feel that it is not a subject to be openly discussed. Thankfully, this is changing.

In many tribal cultures, menarche (the first period) is a time of celebration. It represents an initiation into different roles and responsibilities within the community, and it is celebrated as a community event. In many of these cultures, the fathers create these celebrations. In Western culture, studies show that girls feel that their fathers *should* know they have begun having periods but are not comfortable discussing this with them.

Many ancient cultures had a place for women to go during their time of bleeding, to be relieved of their household responsibilities, to rest and be in the company of other women. Sometimes, such as in early Hebrew tribes, menstruation was seen as an "unclean" time and that was given as the reason for separating the women, but the women themselves generally saw it as a blessing. They wouldn't have traded that time away—spent grooming one another, resting, and sharing stories—for being considered "clean" any day. Anita Diamant, in her book *The Red Tent*, shows beautifully how this time among the women signaled a change in a girl's status within the tribe, once she was able to participate. In this place, spending time with other women, seeing how they made decisions, watching them, listening to their stories, a girl would learn from her elders what it was to be a woman. Also, many of the decisions important to the day-to-day operation of the camps were made there among the women, who generally bled near to the same time each month because they were living without artificial light and therefore close to the moon's cycle. This was also true in Native American tribal culture.

How We Are Mirrored

The time surrounding the blossoming of prepubescence into womanhood is a delicate time in terms of self-image and self-esteem. Girls are moving into new roles and a new status. They are forming their ideas about who they are (and will be) and how they will be received as women during this time. The reflections of the father, who is theoretically a safe male mirror, are critical at puberty. How a girl's bodily changes are viewed and responded to by her father can have a significant effect on what she carries forward into womanhood. I had a client who confided that during her teenage years, her father repeatedly made comments about her being "as graceful as a cow" and told her that "dancing was not for girls like her." This woman went on to be a dancer for several years during her life (maybe in rebellion?), but she always carried within her the feeling that she was clumsy. Many women I have seen in my practice have also told stories of how their fathers' critical attitudes and comments about their changing bodies created a self-consciousness that continues until this day. They have always felt that there is something essentially wrong with them.

Even if a father is supportive of the changes in his daughter's body, it can be an awkward time. Many fathers, as they see their daughters turn into women, begin to feel uncomfortable being physically affectionate with them. They feel it is no longer appropriate. For the girls, however, the message is one of being rejected by their fathers, whom they need more than ever during this time. They internalize a message of wrongness and rejection of their womanhood. These experiences can have lasting effects on a woman's perception of herself.

Going Deeper

Your Menstrual Journey

Let's look at how this information relates to your personal journey. What are your stories of menarche and menstruation? Give some time to the following questions and see what comes through for you.

- What were you told ahead of time about menstruation and sexuality? Were you prepared for the experience? Why or why not?

- At what age did you begin to develop breasts, the first visible signs of developing into a woman? How did you feel about this? Excited? Uncomfortable? Scared? What sort of response did you receive to these changes from your mother, father, friends?

- At what age did you start your first menstrual period? Was this earlier or later than your friends? Did this matter to you?

- What was the experience of your first period like? Where did it happen? Who did you tell? How did you feel?

- How were you anticipating your first period? With excitement or dread? What influenced your feelings about menstruation?

- Was this experience shared with your father or was it kept a secret? What was his response, if shared?

- Did you accept your period as a healthy part of being female or was it a nuisance or a "curse" that you would prefer to live without? If a curse, was there anyone else in your life who may have influenced your perspective?

- Did you receive any teaching from an older woman (mother, grandmother, mother of a friend) about how to care for yourself in a way that honored your cycles as a woman and how to support and reap the benefit of what each part of the cycle brought to you?

- How did your parents respond to your growing sexuality and/or sexual orientation?

- When you look in the mirror now, whose voice do you hear in your head? What is the judgment of this voice about how you look?

- What do you wish was different about your body or appearance? What do you love and accept about your body and appearance?

It is often surprising when we go back and look at the messages, experiences, and people that went into creating the image we have of ourselves in the world as women. For instance, body shaming at an early age or an uncomfortable social or sexual experience just as we are entering the world as young women can have a lifelong impact.

If you noticed in this exploration that the self-concept you formed as a young woman was largely determined by the messages of others, it can be useful to go back and tell yourself the story of what it *would* have been like had you received accurate mirroring or if you had the self-confidence at the time to refute what you were being told and live as yourself. Write down what you can remember about how you thought of yourself. How might your story have been different? Sometimes looking at pictures of yourself at different ages can help to bring up the memories associated with this.

Think of some steps you can take now to align yourself with what you know to be true about yourself and express that. The more we embody what we know or suspect to be a true image of ourselves, the easier it is to truly claim it. We have often been made to fear what might happen or how we might be seen if we embody our desires. Even a few experiences of having that *not* happen can release us from this fear.

Chapter 4

Perimenopause

She is both, hellfire and holy water.
And the flavor you taste depends on
how you treat her.　　—Sneha Pal

T he next big event on the hormonal horizon is the onset of *perimenopause*, the five-to-eight-year period prior to *menopause*. Menopause officially begins after one full year without a menstrual period. During this time, periods often become less regular and most women experience more premenstrual symptoms and menopause-like symptoms, such as hot flashes, night sweats, tender breasts, irritability, and difficulty sleeping. Perimenopause begins what most women think of as menopause. Things are starting to change.

Considering what we know about how beliefs and environment affect our physicality, it should be no surprise that a woman's transition into perimenopause is heavily influenced by her attitudes and beliefs about herself as a woman, her past and current hormone balance and stress levels, and the environment in which she lives. The experiences she has had with older women and the stories she has been told about their menopause also play a large part in how she views this phase of her life. What we expect heavily influences what we will experience.

Our Journey Toward Menopause

We are born with all the egg follicles we will ever have, already nestled in the ovaries of our infant bodies. In addition, we carry a great storehouse of information encoded into all of our cells. The science of epigenetics is showing us that our cells actually store memory in their DNA, and that it is possible for nongenetic information to be passed from parent to child and even into future generations. This is thought to happen through various proteins and other cells that cling to the DNA in a fixed pattern. In other words, your cells might carry imprints from your mother's traumas as well as your own, informing you in nonspecific ways. This opens up the fascinating possibility for us as women of direct ancestral memory, because we each lived in our mother's body as an egg, and our mother lived in her mother's body, and she lived in hers, all the way back in time.

These maternal attitudes and possible traumas that live in our bodies might be triggered into expression as we enter menopause and the unknown that it brings, adding further to any anxieties that might be present. Of course, our mother's overt messages and what she shares of her own experiences more importantly add to the mix.

This legacy carries forward into the future as well if we become mothers, because we pass on these "extras" that have recorded environmental influences, emotions, and attitudes in the DNA we give to our children. Psychologists tell us that we often *recapitulate* (repeat) patterns or even have experiences similar to those of our parents at the same time in our lives as they did. Scientists are now able to tell where generational traumas are coded in the DNA that we pass down to our children.

We not only pass genetic information forward to our children but they continue to live in and inform our bodies as well. Once a woman has carried a child in her body, she continues to carry vestiges of that child for the rest of her life. During a pregnancy, stray cells from the growing baby circulate through a mother's body, most likely to inform her immune system so that it doesn't see the baby as a foreign invader and act to reject it. Scientists have found these fetal cells living and circulating in mothers' bodies decades after their children were born, continuing to inform them. I find this intriguing scientific support for what every mother already knows: our babies are always our babies, even when they are grown up. They are, quite literally, still alive in us and our bodies carry on a cellular conversation with their DNA.

Most women have plenty of egg follicles to last through three to four decades of menstrual cycles and potential pregnancies. As mentioned before, Nature likes plenty of backup. However, as we enter our forties, our usual monthly complement of egg follicles decreases significantly, particularly if we are stressed. We are no longer producing up to twenty follicles per month; we are producing only half that amount or less. When we finally run out of egg follicles and stop having periods, we are considered to be in menopause. For most women, this happens between the ages of forty-eight and fifty-five, with fifty-two being the average. Loss of ovarian function prior to age forty is considered medically to be premature menopause.

As our numbers of egg follicles decrease, our levels of progesterone go down as well, bringing with it all of the symptoms of low progesterone, often beginning with irritability and moodiness. We often feel like we are on a hair trigger. Some women also experience anxiety and difficulty sleeping (progesterone is a calming hormone), tender breasts, increased bloating, and often bleeding irregularities (longer, heavier periods, two "periods" in a month, or an occasional missed period). This is what happens first.

My client Lucy originally came to me because she couldn't tolerate the person she became leading up to and during her period.

"I don't see how my husband stands me," she said. "I am always snapping at him. It is like I am standing outside of my body, watching someone else, watching words come out of my mouth I would *never* ordinarily say. *Everything* irritates me. I can't stop myself and I can't stand myself." We discussed stress levels and nutrients that could help, supported her adrenals with supplements and lifestyle changes, and started her on a little bioidentical progesterone in the second half of her cycle to make up for what she was missing. Things began to even out right away and though her symptoms didn't completely disappear, this allowed her to be more in control of her behavior.

As we continue toward menopause, our complement of egg follicles gets very low, and our levels of estrogen begin to drop as well. At this time, many women begin to experience hot flashes, night sweats, sleeplessness, thinning skin and hair, and a decrease in sexual desire. Depending on the number of egg follicles remaining and a woman's stress levels, these symptoms may start to appear five to eight years before she actually goes through menopause, which begins after one year of missed periods.

During the last two to three years before menopause, it is very common to miss several periods and then start back up again; or if one ovary runs low in eggs first, to miss every other period. (Our ovaries generally tend to alternate each month for ovulation.) When you think about how the menstrual cycle beats the rhythm of our physical and emotional lives as women, even if we are unconscious of it, it should be no surprise how disruptive it can be when this rhythm changes. It can be a very confusing time.

The Role of the Adrenal Glands

The symptoms of perimenopause are made worse when stress levels are high, because it is the job of the adrenal glands and fat cells to take over hormone production when the ovaries wind down.

Your stress gets all of your body's attention. Nature always prioritizes survival over reproduction, so sex-hormone levels (estrogen, progesterone, and testosterone) will always be lower when stress is present. All of the precursors for making your sex hormones will instead go toward making stress hormones, and what sex hormones you have left will often be turned into stress hormones.

During perimenopause, many women also start to exhibit symptoms of adrenal exhaustion and begin to show signs of high blood pressure, unstable blood sugar, high cholesterol, foggy brain, weight gain, and decreasing stamina. Most women think they are just "getting old," and there is nothing they can do about it. But if you look at how all the threads in your bodily universe are connected, there is actually a very simple reason for it and it is definitely within your power to reverse these symptoms. The answer lies with the adrenal glands and how they work.

If you remember, the adrenal glands are all about survival for the body, and they mount what we call the fight-or-flight response to stress. Every time our body goes into fight-or-flight, four things happen:

- the liver empties its emergency stores of sugar and fat into the bloodstream (to give the body quick energy);

- the blood pressure goes up (to push the blood deeper into the muscles to give them more strength);

- the blood is shunted from the brain to the extremities (to give the body more power); and

- the immune system is suppressed (so that if you are injured, you can continue to fight or run instead of being stopped dead by a huge inflammatory response).

If someone has been living with a lot of stress and their body is frequently in the fight-or-flight state (which typically lasts two to three hours), then they have spent a lot of time in a state of high blood sugar, high blood pressure, less blood to the brain, and a suppressed immune system. It is no wonder that the diseases that we suffer from most as middle- and older-aged adults are diabetes, high blood pressure, depression, obesity, and autoimmune syndromes.

Many women also find around the time of perimenopause and menopause that they are suddenly low in thyroid hormone. They are told they have *hypothyroidism* (low thyroid), and most commonly this is caused by Hashimoto's syndrome, an autoimmune disease where the body begins to attack its own thyroid gland.

The state of the adrenals has a huge effect on how well the thyroid functions. Our thyroid gland can be working fine and yet we can still have symptoms of low thyroid if the adrenals are exhausted and our cortisol levels are low. We need adequate levels of cortisol for the thyroid to convert the hormone thyroxine (T4), which the thyroid makes, to liothyronine (T3), which is the form that the tissues in the body actually use.

This process of converting T4 to T3 is mediated by the enzyme thyroid peroxidase. If the body does not have enough cortisol because of exhausted adrenals, that enzyme cannot help the thyroid make that conversion and we end up without enough T3, or bioactive thyroid hormone, to do its work in the body. The result is low energy, slow metabolism, dry skin and hair, brittle nails, constipation, and sometimes depression. In fact, if you look at the package insert on any thyroid medication, it will tell you not to start thyroid medication until you address any low levels of cortisol.

Often I have found in my practice that when a woman's tests show low thyroid and low adrenal function, just treating the adrenals often balances out the thyroid and there is no need to start thyroid medication at all. This is a good thing, because once someone starts taking thyroid hormone, it is rare to be able to stop taking it.

As you can see, the adrenals are like the base of the pyramid in the body, holding everything else up; again, survival before everything else as far as Mother Nature is concerned! So, for an easier perimenopause and menopause, it is important to take your stress seriously and to support your adrenals! A salivary adrenal function panel that shows your cortisol levels when you wake in the morning, at noon, just before dinner, and at bedtime will show if your adrenal rhythm and cortisol levels are adequate. Treatment will be different, depending on which values are low.

Since the adrenals have everything to do with energy, clarity, metabolism, and a strong immune system, you will feel better in the short term and create an easier menopausal transition in the long term if you take your stress seriously and address any adrenal insufficiency you might have. There are several lifestyle adjustments that can be made to support the adrenals, which I will discuss in chapter 6, "Caring for Ourselves at Midlife."

How the Body Sees Stress

Given how intricate the connection is between our adrenal glands, our sex hormone levels, and the stability of those levels, it is useful to look at the role stress has played in our lives. You have already done a little inquiry into the stress levels of your mother during her pregnancy with you and that of your early home life. How did your stress levels evolve as you started school; interacted with your peers; had to compete for grades, jobs, and intimate partners? Remember, good stress or bad stress—it is all just stress to the body.

The pace alone of current lifestyles is stressful to the body. Often, contrary to what we might think, the more successful we are in cultural terms (status, jobs, our personal lives), the greater our physical stress. Just the fact that we are expected to be available almost twenty-four hours a day by phone, fax, email, and instant

messaging is stressful, as it leaves no islands of quiet for contempla-
tion, regeneration, and renewal for the body.

A woman may love her life. She may be up at 5:30 a.m., fueled
by her morning latte, hit the gym, head to a fast-paced job she
loves that keeps her interested and going all day, then leave work
for a party or dinner with her friends or lover. She's in bed at
11:30 p.m. or midnight and has plans for an exciting, fun-filled
weekend. In fact, this is what we are told we should *aspire* to by
the marketing gurus. Yet this woman will suffer almost the same
stress to her body as a woman who works two jobs, takes care of
children without help, suffers from financial stress, or has an abu-
sive husband. They are both under significant stress—one positive
and one negative. The difference would be that the stress of the
downtrodden woman could reach the cellular level, modifying her
DNA much like trauma does.

In fact, the first woman in this story may not consider herself
stressed at all. She loves her life and lives it fully, fueled by adrenaline and caffeine, which *feels* great. A little adrenaline into the mix
makes us feel alert, smart, energetic, and clear, because if we were
actually *in* a fight-or-flight situation—say, running from a bear
in the woods—we would need those heightened senses to survive.
The happy woman will only be suffering from physical stress, but
she will have the positive effect to her body of loving her life. The
downtrodden woman, oppressed by her stress, has that negative
feedback to her body in addition to the physical stress. In both
cases, the stress to the adrenals leads to hormone imbalance, and
this creates a downward spiral.

Often, women who come to me because of perimenopausal
and menopausal symptoms write on their intake forms that their
stress levels are "not that bad." Many of them have lived and
worked for much of their lives in cities as writers, artists, business
executives, or entrepreneurs. They do not rate their lives as very

stressful because they love what they do. However, when we look for downtime—regeneration time—it is not there. They are getting to bed late, getting up early, running all day on not enough food and too much caffeine, meeting deadlines, engaging in bicoastal and international traveling, and attending social engagements. The woman living a life where she feels oppressed or overburdened *knows* she is stressed. These women often do not.

When we test the adrenals of these women with *positive* stress, we find them to be every bit as exhausted as the women with the nine-to-five job, household responsibilities, and children. Both women are functioning on too little sleep, not enough nourishment, and no downtime.

We can live like this and not feel it for a while if we are young and have some reserves, but eventually our bodies have to pay the price. Much like a bank account, we can use up the biochemicals our bodies need and not feel it too much as long as we have some left to draw on in emergencies. But if we continue to spend unnecessarily, we deplete our reserves and suffer the consequences of overdraft. And when that happens, it often comes all at once and seemingly out of the blue. We are adaptable creatures, and after a while, almost any level of stress begins to seem like the new normal, so we may not notice that we're depleting our energy stores. We are just meeting the requirements of each day as it comes.

Evaluating Your Stress

So, let's begin by making a "good for me/bad for me" list. Take some quiet time and go somewhere you can hear your own thoughts. Turn off your cell phone, take a breath, and look at your life with a bold eye. Begin by making a thorough list of everything in your life that nourishes you and brings you pleasure. Is there any way to get more of that? Anything you would like to add to the list that is not there?

Next, make a list of everything in your life that takes your energy (whether it seems worthy, positive or not) and doesn't give anything back. Study this list carefully. What can you let go of here? This list might contain friends, family, activities, or long-standing commitments. What is still alive for you in present time? You must find a way to let go of the things that suck your vital force and give nothing back.

Some of these things, people, and activities will be easy to identify as irrelevant to your current life. Others will be more difficult to tease out. Is a friendship more of a habit than a true give-and-take relationship? Do you continue with an activity only because you feel you would "look bad" if you dropped it?

Women can easily fall into the trap of needing to be needed; however, others can generally be found to take over those responsibilities if we move on. This is a good time to look at whether your need to be needed is keeping a person or organization in a dependent mode, and might actually be holding *them* back. Is there an unconscious dynamic of having another dependent on you that makes you feel safer? As I said, look with a bold eye. Tell yourself the truth.

You also likely have people, activities, and commitments that take a lot of your energy but either carry some reward or for which you are responsible, and cannot change. This category may include family, a much-needed job, or activities for which you have timed commitments that haven't run out. In cases like these, it becomes necessary to set new boundaries.

Here is an example. My client Ruth was being driven crazy by multiple daily calls from her mother, who would complain endlessly about her problems and why her life was miserable. Ruth was an only child, and her mother was a widow with few friends and activities to take the burden off of Ruth. No amount of Ruth's attempted problem-solving, empathizing, or giving tempered her mother's behavior. This was a major stressor in Ruth's life, taking up most of her "free" time and almost all of her psychic space and emotional energy. She felt she was going under and didn't know what to do. Ruth felt responsible to care for her mother, but this was more than she could handle. She had told her mother this, but to no avail. Ruth and I discussed the possibility of shifting her mother's behavior by setting some boundaries, in order for Ruth to feel a sense of control over her own life.

She came back to her next visit a month later, much more relaxed and having found a solution. Ruth stated that she had told her mother, lovingly but firmly, that she could only be available to her on the phone for fifteen minutes a day, in the early evening. During that time, she would be happy to listen to anything her mother wished to tell her, but when the fifteen minutes were up, she was going to hang up. She had practiced this approach over the intervening few weeks, consistently and without anger, giving her mother all of her attention for fifteen minutes and then calmly saying, "Our time is up for today; I'm going to hang up now," and doing it.

Her mother fought her at first and tried calling back, but Ruth stuck with her plan. The behavior stopped after about a week, and Ruth and her mother settled into a rhythm of nightly fifteen-minute phone calls, where Ruth's mother had her full attention during that time and the rest of Ruth's evening was her own.

Going Deeper

Exploring the Stress in Our Lives

Now that you have some experience evaluating the current stress in your life, take a look at how stress has showed up in your life previous to this and how it might have affected your menstrual rhythms or your perimenopause.

- What were your parents' expectations of you growing up? Did they run a "tight ship" or were things relaxed around the home?

- Did your parents allow you to be a kid or were you expected to be a miniature adult and behave at all times, have good manners, and not cause "trouble"?

- How fully did you meet your parents' expectations? Did you feel that you were competent or always somehow lacking? How has this affected you going forward?

- What was your elementary school experience like? Were you well accepted by teachers and peers or did you feel like an outsider? Why?

- What about middle school/junior high school? Were you accepted, rejected, lonely, scared?

- What about high school? As your workload and social pressures increased, did you feel performance anxiety or were you comfortable in your school environment?

- Follow this through to any higher education, the job hunt, or the workplace. Where did the stress come from? Was it time management? Feelings of competence? Feelings of belonging or not belonging? Financial stress? Feelings of safety or not being safe? Relationships with family, lovers, or coworkers? What areas of your life tend to be stressful? How do these relate to your childhood home, if at all?

- Have you experienced a significant medical illness during your life? At what age? Did it pass or is this a chronic condition that you must still address?

Now take a look at how stress might have affected your hormonal balance during these various phases of your life.

- At the age your period started, was there more or less stress in your life? What kinds of stress?

- Was your period regular right from the start or did it take a couple of years of starts and stops before regulating?

- What were your periods like? Were they comfortable or did you have a lot of cramping, bloating, and premenstrual symptoms?

- Did your periods remain regular or was there a time that you stopped bleeding, became less regular, or your symptoms of discomfort increased? What were the stressors in your life at that time?

- If you tried to become pregnant, was this easy for you or did you have a difficult time conceiving? What was happening in other areas of your life at the time?

- At what age did you begin to experience perimenopausal or menopausal symptoms? When did you begin to skip periods?

- What do you notice in terms of symptoms, energy level, or ability to sleep when there are more stressors present in your life? What might you do to address this?

Being exposed to the material in this chapter and doing this self-exploration can bring with it a sense of anxiety, because it might feel too overwhelming or "too late" to do anything about the stress in your life. You might already be having menopausal symptoms and feel that nothing you do now will be powerful enough to change that. You might feel trapped in a situation that does not allow you to reduce your stress. I want to reassure you that even small changes, such as changing your bedtime, can have a significant ripple effect.

Likewise, there are things that we might be aware of under the surface that won't come to clarity until we really sit down and focus on looking for them. It is very easy just to think that we are prone to illness or accidents or that timing is always wrong for us—any number of stories we might tell ourselves based on our past experiences. Yet when we go back and look at *what else was happening around us* in our lives and make the connections in terms of timing, a different story emerges.

Making a time line is very effective for this kind of investigation. Get out a big piece of paper and draw a line across it. Starting with your birth, mark major stressors and the age they happened—and then go back and fill in your body's responses to these. Or mark your body's expressions (illness, injury, symptoms) at various ages and times of your life and then look for the concurrent stressors, whichever way is easiest for you.

Now that you know that the body sees *good stress* and *bad stress* as the same, you might be able to make some new connections. In whatever way is most intuitive to you, make these connections. Write them down and keep these reflections somewhere that you can look at them often, and add to them when you think of something. See what bubbles up. Note any insights that arise. The simple act of being able to reframe things in this way can help you shift your perspective and begin to change the underlying stress in your life. Once you know something, you can't unknow it.

Chapter 5

Menopause

She remembered who she was and
the game changed.   —Lalah Delia

S
o, we have arrived at menopause. We know something about the path that brought us here. Why is menopause something we fear? I think it is largely because what we hear about menopause has been pulled out of context and only one part of it has been highlighted for us—the symptoms. We feel that menopause is something that *happens to* us; we have no control over how it unfolds and no input into where it goes. We don't see it as part of our life's continuum. Because it is taken out of the context of the rest of our lives, it makes no sense.

Our medical community focuses on the symptoms of menopause because they are oriented toward "fixing" things, and this is something they can attempt to fix. But menopause *isn't* something to be fixed. It is the way Nature prepares us for our next phase of life. We dread menopause because by and large, the stories we hear are negative. Nature did not intend it to be so. It is, in fact, the time when we begin to bear the fruit of our lives. When our reproductive years are over, Nature's purpose leans more toward integration and civilization building; succession, passing on what we have gathered and learned; and mentoring those who come after us. It should be no surprise that the hormonal shifts during menopause support these tasks. This integration happens physically, emotionally, and in terms of our consciousness and evolution as a species. There is much that is in our power to control.

Many women are confused about when menopause actually begins and ends. I often hear women say, "Oh, I already did menopause. I am past that." However, as we discussed in earlier chapters, most women have their most intense symptoms before menopause begins, in perimenopause. Menopause itself actually begins after there have been no periods for a year and we can safely assume that we will not conceive a child. Being menopausal doesn't end. We are menopausal, or some would say postmenopausal, for the rest of our lives.

Many women go through two or three years of having a period here and there before they stop for good. They think menopause has finally arrived and then they will have one, two, or three periods in a row. The hormones come in spits and spurts during this transition out of the reproductive years, just as they did coming into it. Though less likely, the menopausal transition can also happen as it did for my client Sarah: you can be regular every month and then one month your period just doesn't come, and never comes again. There is no way to predict how it will be for you, though stress plays a big part in this, as we have seen.

Once menopause is firmly established (you have had no periods for a full year), the picture looks somewhat different for each woman, depending on her physical health, relationships, environment, stress levels, and beliefs about what this stage of life should look like. For some women, the transition is easy. For others, it is life-changing in a negative way. Much of how we experience menopause has to do with our perceptions and beliefs about aging and our visions for what the second half of life will be like. The change is emotional, physical, and what I would call spiritual, in terms of changes to our consciousness.

Your Physical Journey

As we have seen, hormone balance and how it informs the brain is a fluid process with different goals at different stages of life. We are somewhat androgynous in our early years as we develop our physical body and our brain's capacities. We polarize for the purposes of reproduction, when Nature's prime directive for us is to make replacements for ourselves and continue the species. When our reproductive years are over, Nature's purpose leans more toward creativity, integration of what we have learned, and passing this to those who come after. And just as in earlier transitions, the hormonal shifts during menopause support us in doing this.

The form of estrogen that is in highest concentration during our reproductive years is estradiol. Estradiol stimulates the part of our brain that makes us want to go out and make babies and nurture everything in sight. It has us cooing over babies in the supermarket and scanning men for their genetic potential, even if we are happily paired. This is also the estrogen that makes it a little easier for us to be a doormat to our mate and our children, to do more than is humanly possible for our family (work full time, cook, clean, shop, chauffeur, nurture) while putting ourselves at the bottom of our own to-do list. It is as if we are in a hormonal trance, induced by Mother Nature, to ensure the survival of the species.

After menopause, the primary circulating estrogen is estriol, which stimulates a different part of our brain. Estriol lights up our creative centers. Women at midlife often move toward wanting to write that book, dance that dance, paint that painting, start a business, or take on a cause—the seeds of which were often present when they were younger, before surges of estradiol turned them into baby-making machines. It should come as no surprise, then, that estriol levels are very high in the body when we are being the most literally creative we will ever be—when we are growing a baby inside of us.

For both women and men, as we enter the integrative years, hormones move from the male/female poles to a more neutral balance. In men, testosterone levels drop and estrogen levels rise (creating the "beer bellies" and "man boobs" we are so fond of joking about). In women, testosterone levels rise as estrogen drops, sometimes creating more facial and body hair and often bringing our anger to the surface.

The issues that cause this anger may have been present for decades, but the drop in estradiol (which encourages us to smooth everything over for the sake of nurturing) and the rise in testosterone (which is associated with more anger and aggression) often lifts the lid off of suppressed issues and memories and brings them to the fore. For many women and their partners, this can be confusing and scary. Though anger is an accepted and sometimes even admired trait in men if it gets them where they want to go in the world, our culture doesn't support anger or aggressiveness in women. An angry woman is often seen as a bitch or, at best, overreactive.

The women (and their partners) who move forward whole into the next phase of life do not become mired in guilt or allow themselves to be forced back into more docile molds. They see what their anger is there to teach them about—what has been suppressed. They are open to exploring, claiming, and releasing the past and catching up to the present.

The physical changes that most women go through take place in several arenas. The skin becomes thinner and drier and more easily shows lines and wrinkles. The body accumulates an extra five to seven pounds, mostly around the middle, to assist with hormone production. Muscle tone diminishes with a consequent sense of "sagging" thighs, belly, and upper arms that used to be more toned. If we are caught up to present time in our lives and living from an authentic place, we can mourn the passing of our youthful bodies and begin to appreciate the new velvety texture to our skin and the shape that declares we have made a passage. For those of us who have been taught that our value is tied to our youthful looks, or who continue to cling to outdated versions of ourselves rather than mourning and releasing the passing of those, menopause can be the hell that so many describe.

I have many clients for whom the change in skin texture that comes with menopause is so distressing that it makes them forget about their own safety: "I can't stand the fact that my skin is thinner. I'm losing muscle tone. I'm sagging. That's not okay. I will take as high a dose of hormones as it takes to change it back." Or "I'm getting this fat around my belly. I've never had a belly! I'm hardly eating *anything* and I exercise *every* day for two hours and it's still there." Or "My breasts are sagging. How can I stop it? Do I have to get implants? I don't want to, but I can't stand this! Help me!" You get the picture. Most of us have had similar thoughts, even if we don't express them. Change is hard.

We live in a culture that deifies youth, and many women in menopause now were raised to place their primary value on their looks. Given our very narrow cultural view of what is considered attractive, menopause—with its attendant changes in body shape, skin texture, hair volume, and energy level—can be a nightmare for these women.

Being Proactive

Some women, as they approach menopause and begin to experience changes, want to be proactive and educate themselves as to how best to prepare for this next stage, what to expect, and how to support themselves. These women may have positive menopause models in their lives, or they may have seen their mothers go through hell and they are determined that they are "not going there." These women are generally health conscious and like to be prepared, to "take care of business" in their lives.

One such person is my client Patti. She came into my office in her midforties, before she was experiencing any symptoms, and said, "I want to be prepared." Since she was not in the throes of destabilizing symptoms and in search of "fixes," and since she wasn't feeling desperate, we were able to take the time to explore her earlier hormonal life and her models for what was coming. We looked at her patterns of stress, and she identified some places she could change that trajectory. Her testing showed that like most women in their forties, her progesterone was low, so she started a little bit of bioidentical progesterone in the second half of her cycle. She put lifestyle changes in place that encouraged a balance of active time and downtime, normalized her sleep patterns, and optimized her nutrition.

As she continued to move through her forties and entered menopause, Patti did not experience the debilitating symptoms that many women do. Her periods were a little less regular, but she sailed right through menopause without hot flashes, sleep disruption, irritability, or fatigue. She had built up the base of the pyramid, the adrenals, and the benefits of being proactive were evident: she was able to see the path before her, to know what causes menopausal changes and what to expect, so that they didn't take her by surprise. She was able to normalize the process and even avoid many of the symptoms by working early to bring her body into balance. Things didn't feel out of control.

Many symptoms that are natural to experience in the menopausal years—hot flashes, heart palpitations, sleeplessness, thinning hair, painful sex, depression, aching joints—would be considered signs of illness at any other time of life, and many women truly fear that they have become ill and that they are in danger of dying. They see it as the beginning of a long downhill slide.

Most uncomfortable menopausal symptoms are somewhat temporary; they wax and wane and usually disappear within a few years if stress levels are under control. If a woman is not aware of the transitory nature of her symptoms, she may feel that this is the "new normal" and fall into despair. For instance, sleep deprivation is a bona fide method of torture. It changes brain chemistry and causes us to slip the tether of reality, preventing us from properly interpreting social cues and causing reactivity and irritability. If it goes on long enough, we exhaust our adrenals (because we're not supplying the deep uninterrupted sleep the adrenals need to repair themselves) and our hormonal scaffold collapses even further.

So, being prepared for what might come and arming ourselves with the tools and tactics to prevent much of it is a good strategy, when we have the presence of mind and can carve out the time in our lives to do it. I encourage you to think ahead, address your stress, and find someone who can help you balance your hormones, if needed, *before* things start to feel significantly imbalanced.

Not every woman has the extra "brain space" to be proactive. Many women are barely getting through their to-do lists in life as it is; they are pretty much just reacting to whatever shows up each day. These women find themselves in the middle of menopause before they have given it any thought, and come to see me in various states of concern, despair, or determination to find out what is happening and what can be done. The deeper someone is into a downward physical spiral, the longer it will take to unravel. But if a woman will work with her body and be consistent, she will come back to balance. In my experience, we must engage with the work—there is no magic pill.

Your Emotional Journey

Women's responses to the changes of menopause are as varied as the women themselves, and women on every part of the continuum come through my door. There is no good or bad way to engage this part of our lives. We are where we are, and *anywhere* we are is where we take our first step forward in our journey toward balance and vibrant health. Remember, "you can pull any thread and unravel the universe." You are *always* on the path, wherever you are, and any positive step you take will have a ripple effect outward to everything else.

Unfortunately, our culture views the menopausal transition and the menopausal years as a time of loss. Once we enter this part of life, we have "lost" our youth, "lost" our looks, "lost" our appeal and our value as women. I have also found that, just as with pregnancy, most of the stories women tell one another about this time of life are the horror stories.

This always struck me as rather sad, that we as women always seem to educate other women with negative stories. We rarely hear women telling about what a wonderful pregnancy they had or how empowering labor and birthing was for them. We hear about the pain, the intervention, the time when the baby almost died; everything about how the body did *not* work as it was meant to. The same is true for menopause. We are not given models of the potential empowerment of this time of life, only the downside. I have often wondered why this is, and I can only conclude that women are unconsciously still trying to work through their own trauma when sharing stories like these; otherwise, there is no benefit that I can see to doing so. It highlights the lack of opportunities that we have as women in this culture to tell our stories and heal our traumas, and it perpetuates the cultural myth that the path of a woman's life is fraught with danger and pain.

Add to that the fact that women whose lives were centered around the needs of children and family find their nests empty and no longer feel their purpose as clearly, nor do their families understand this shift. Sometimes families feel abandoned or partners react with anger when a woman no longer focuses entirely on them. To these women, this time of transition can feel like being dropped down in the middle of the jungle without a compass and told to find your way home. It is no surprise really that even in my mother's generation, women were sometimes institutionalized or diagnosed as mentally ill just because they were going through menopause and no one understood the cause of their symptoms and changes in affect, or how to help them.

These days, with women delaying childbearing (often well into their thirties or early forties) to pursue a career or because they haven't found the appropriate partner, many women find themselves going through menopause with young children to mother. They don't have the hormonal support for raising young children that they would have had earlier in life and their adrenals are tired, making physical exhaustion, weight gain, and irritability even more likely to occur. Often these women feel like they are failing as mothers because they don't have the help of the more nurturing hormones that younger women do, and they have begun to want things for themselves again. They are beginning to dream of their next creative stage of life.

It is important to ask for help if we need it. It is a good time of life for *many* reasons to find a good friend, a therapist, or someone to listen, to help us orient; and it is *critical* that we talk with our partners. They are quite often very confused, and will take things personally. To engage with your partner during this changing time and look forward *together* to what you want to create as a couple is very powerful. In the case of male partners, they are often going through changes themselves that are not as culturally recognized, and we all tend to want to blame someone or something else when things get confusing and scary. Make them your companion in this journey, not someone standing on the outside looking in.

Going Deeper

Your Stories of Menopause

A woman's attitudes toward aging and her pictures of what the second half of life will be like heavily influence the experience she will actually have in menopause. Through your self-inquiry in earlier chapters of this book, you have begun to have a sense of how you relate to being female, what the early messages were that you received from family and friends about womanhood, and how that changed as your body began to proclaim your femaleness in more visible ways.

When the monthly cycle ceases for good, the hormonal support for nurturing others diminishes somewhat as well. If we have *not* been caring for ourselves up to this point in time, our menopausal symptoms will be worse and we will see, with no filters, what it is that is not working for us in our lives. In some ways, it is like removing a pair of blinders. We come out of the hormonal trance and see where we truly are. For some women, this is enough to send them running in the other direction. Many women, though, see it as an opportunity to take stock, to reorient, and to move forward with fresh energy and creativity. Which of these questions calls to you?

- At what age did you first begin to have menopausal symptoms? Were you expecting them? What were they?

- Which symptoms caused you the most concern? Why? Were you concerned that you were sick or something was wrong?

- How old were you when you ceased having periods? Was it something you welcomed?

- What were your experiences with other women going through menopause? Your mother? Friends?

- What stories were you told about this time of life? What were your expectations?

- Did you see menopause in terms of loss or liberation? What influenced your viewpoint?

- What has been the response of your partner and friends to the fact that you are now menopausal?

- Has the way you express yourself creatively changed? If so, how?

- Do you have a close circle of support? If not, how might you create this in your life?

As mentioned before, menopause is a crossroads at which women generally decide to move forward and thrive or begin to diminish. This is a decision that comes not once but again and again, and in different areas of our being. We may think we are handling everything well emotionally and yet find that we just can't gather the energy to deal with our stress or our body's symptoms of aging. We might be fit and engaged with our family and community and yet find ourselves without a partner and begin to give up on having that. If that is important to us, it might not feel worth moving forward and continuing to try in other areas of our lives. Moving forward toward a positive menopause is a process of saying *YES* over and over again; falling down and getting up. It is the direction we move in, and the fact that we *continue* to move, that makes the difference.

In your explorations thus far, you have likely uncovered some areas of your life that you would like to investigate further and possibly shift into alignment with what feels authentic to you now. You might wish to identify the areas that you feel you need to address in order to come into present time.

Once you have identified them, what might the first step be to bring yourself into alignment with what you desire? It might be having a conversation with someone in particular, letting go of something that no longer resonates with you, or committing to something new. You might feel it would be useful to work with a therapist or particular healing modality.

If you are symptomatic and feel it would be helpful to you to stabilize before attempting anything else, find a practitioner who works with bioidentical hormones and take a saliva test to look at your hormone levels and adrenal function. If you do not know of a practitioner in your area, you can call a local compounding pharmacist and ask them for a referral. Compounding pharmacists work closely with these practitioners and generally know who women like to work with and who gets good results with their clients.

Whatever the steps you wish to take, gather your allies and make a commitment to yourself and others. Having support and good mirroring always adds to your chances for success.

Chapter 6

Caring for Ourselves
at Midlife

With every act of self-care, your authentic self gets
stronger, and the critical, fearful mind gets weaker.
Every act of self-care is a powerful declaration:
I am on my side. —Susan Weiss Berry

A
s we have seen, lifestyle and the state of our adrenals can
have a huge impact on our menopause. This time of our lives
can be a wake-up call to begin to assess what our bodies
need and how we are living, and a prompt to take better care of
ourselves. It is kind of like the old adage of the frog—if dropped
into boiling water, it will jump right out; but if you put it in
lukewarm water and slowly increase the temperature to boiling,
it just keeps on adapting and dies as a result.

Many of us have been slowly adapting to more and more stress
over the years, to the point that it now seems normal to us. Ways
of being we could tolerate and adapt to, or even enjoyed, when
younger just do not work for us anymore. I have had many women
tell me that they used to be able to go out for drinks every night
after work and stay up late with no lasting effects, or run on
adrenaline and coffee with four or five hours of sleep. Their bodies
no longer do well with these behaviors, but they find it hard to
change them. Some say they resist changing because it makes them

feel old, or it feels like a last rebellion. For others, it is as if these behaviors form a kind of scaffolding that holds them up. They are just making it day to day and are too busy to think about it.

It should come as no surprise that the lifestyle adjustments that support the adrenals will also help to prevent and lessen the symptoms of menopause. Healthy adrenal glands will support overall health and strengthen the immune system, as well as support good hormone balance, since your body will not be turning your sex hormones into stress hormones. (Remember, Nature will always prioritize survival over reproduction.) Instead, the adrenals can do their intended job of supplying the hormones for the second half of life. There are some very simple things you can put into place now that will make a huge difference in terms of how you experience menopause, whether or not you are already having symptoms.

Old habits can be very difficult to break, however, and new habits difficult to form. The brain is a very habit-forming organ, and it can take six weeks to six months of a new behavior (depending on the individual) before the brain creates the new pathways that support maintaining a new habit.

Women in the second half of life benefit tremendously from creating rhythms in their lives. This both helps to conserve energy in the body and helps the brain to form new habits. The amount of energy we have available to use on a daily basis is created by a delicate balance between building up the biochemicals that we need for our energy and the running of bodily processes and using up these resources. Establishing a rhythm to your life allows your body to anticipate at what time of day you will be eating, exercising, or sleeping and therefore have the appropriate amount of energy ready for you at the right time. If, on the other hand, you are random about your activities, your body must have a lot of energy available at all times because it never knows what is going to be asked of it. Generating this energy, to keep you in a constant state of readiness, makes it more likely that you will run low.

Again, the metaphor of a bank account is useful here. The money you have available to use for your daily spending is dependent on what you have in the bank. If you use more than you save, or if you spend needlessly, you will eventually be overdrawn and not have what you need on hand. So, it makes sense to conserve and not to spend needlessly. It is the same with our energy stores. We can take supplements until the cows come home, but if we are not making changes to our lifestyle and we are using up everything that we put in every day, we will never make progress. Creating a rhythm can make a huge difference in helping you conserve while trying to heal.

Following are some basic lifestyle adjustments you can put into place that will make a big difference to your adrenal health, your immune system, and your overall well-being. I have had clients for whom just changing one made all the difference with their menopausal symptoms. Remember, it is all connected and one change will have a ripple effect.

Sleep

Eight hours of deep, uninterrupted sleep every night is one of the most critical foundations for good health, especially in the second half of life, and it is the holy grail for a lot of menopausal women. It is one of the first things to go as the adrenals become fatigued, as we enter midlife and our hormone balance begins to shift. This is because cortisol (the primary stress hormone) and sleep disruption go hand in hand.

There is a natural rhythm to normal cortisol production during the day. Our highest levels are thirty minutes after awakening—the rising level of cortisol in our bloodstream is partly what wakes us up in the morning—then there is a steep drop around noon, and then it slowly tapers off until bedtime. Our lowest levels are between 10 and 10:30 p.m., which encourages the body toward sleep. However, if we stay up much later than this (which most people in our culture do), then our cortisol levels will begin to rise again; our body will mount fight-or-flight in order to give us a second wind and the energy with which to stay up and do what we need to do. High cortisol levels make sleep much more difficult when we *do* go to bed.

Many of us also watch TV or spend time on the computer right before bed, either to relax or because it is our only time to catch up with email and other tasks. For those of us with children or who are working from home, it might be the only quiet time we have to ourselves all day, to get things done. But watching TV and, to a lesser extent, being on the computer will raise cortisol levels slightly, enough to make a difference in our sleep. While watching TV—lying on the couch and staring at a screen—may feel relaxing, something very different is happening in the body. Studies have shown that the brain receives information while we're watching TV, as if the body were actually experiencing it. This information bypasses the part of the brain that analyzes and filters the information. Particularly with television, and the frequent cuts from scene to scene every few seconds, cortisol levels are raised and create a mild fight-or-flight response in the body, even if we don't feel the adrenaline. Television stations and advertisers design programming purposefully to raise cortisol levels, heighten our senses, and keep us riveted, the way we are during fight-or-flight. In addition, the blue spectrum light emitted from computers stimulates the same centers in the brain that tell us it is time to wake up in the morning.

When we go to bed with higher cortisol levels, we will have difficulty falling asleep or we will find that we awaken after just a couple of hours. Even if we fall right to sleep, the sleep is not as deep and therefore not as restorative. High cortisol levels also make it easier to be awakened.

If you think about it, this makes sense. If you had been fighting a bear in the woods all day, your cortisol levels would be elevated when you lay down to sleep. And even if you were exhausted, you wouldn't get a deep, restful sleep. You would be sleeping with one eye open to see if that bear was coming back. In that state of higher cortisol, you would be primed for adrenaline so that if you *did* hear anything, you could be up and out of there like a shot.

So, when sleeping with higher levels of cortisol, we are in a lighter state of sleep, more aware of our environment and more easily brought to consciousness by little things—our bladder, our partner snoring, the cat on the bed or at the door, even stimulating dreams. And if we are startled awake, and there is a further surge of adrenaline, we will likely toss and turn and have our mind circling around things for up to two hours before we can fall back to sleep again—even if we are exhausted—because, remember, fight-or-flight lasts for two to three hours each time it is triggered. Having to get up with an alarm, before our body awakens naturally, compounds this problem.

The adrenals do their repair in the deepest stage of sleep. If we are staying up past 10 or 10:30 p.m., then we will slowly and consistently get less and less of the repair and regeneration our adrenals need, and we will continue to burn up more and more of our existing biochemicals, leading to fatigued adrenals. Add to that the stresses of our normal day-to-day modern life—caring for family, increased stresses of work, relationship problems, physical illness, financial crises—and we can see why women arrive at midlife with compromised adrenals that are unable to support the work of the menopausal transition.

Research also suggests that lack of sleep is related to weight gain, depressed immune system, and psychological depression. Think back to the four things that happen when the body goes into fight-or-flight—elevated blood sugar, elevated blood pressure, less blood to the brain, and a suppressed immune system—and the symptoms make sense. These are all related to stressed adrenals.

So, it is a good practice in any case, but especially if you are trying to heal your adrenals, to head for the barn by 10 p.m. and be asleep by 10:30 p.m. Allow a minimum of thirty minutes between TV and bedtime (one hour is better). If you have a show you are wedded to, record it for viewing earlier in the day or evening.

Have a ritual—a shower, reading for a half hour, yoga, tea—that lets your body know that it is time for bed. If you usually go to bed much later but have a real energy dip earlier in the evening, say at 9:30 p.m., try going with the dip and see what happens. For instance, many people fall asleep on the couch in front of the TV or while reading. After a couple of hours of sleep, they get up, brush their teeth, and go to bed. But that activity has interrupted their sleep and will keep them from sleeping as deeply once they go to bed.

If you don't have an earlier energy dip and usually stay up much later, try shaving fifteen minutes a week off of your bedtime, until you hit 10 or 10:30 p.m., so that the change comes slowly. If you try to do it all at once, you will probably end up staring at the ceiling for hours, frustrated. If going to bed earlier feels like punishment to you, then just think of it as a three- or four-month healing phase. But chances are, once you see the changes that come with getting quantity and quality sleep, you will want to continue. I have had so many women in my practice floored by what a huge difference changing their bedtime made in their lives. As much as possible, allow yourself to sleep until you awaken naturally, without an alarm.

Nutrition

It is not in the scope of this book to go deeply into dietary requirements and the various regimens touted these days. However, it is my belief that there is no one right diet for everyone. Different people just feel better and function better, maintain weight and vitality better, on different kinds of diets. Our oldest systems of medicine (Traditional Chinese Medicine, Ayurveda) recognize that we have different body types and temperaments and that each of them thrives under slightly different conditions. You can find scientific data to back up almost any approach to eating these days, and there are endless arguments among the diet gurus as to which is best.

It has been determined that there are three basic gut types, based on our genetics, and each with its own ecosystem. Some people feel physically better when the majority of their food is vegetable carbohydrate and a smaller percentage is protein and fat. Others do better on high-protein, high-fat diets with very few carbohydrates. Others fall somewhere in the middle. It should be no surprise that the environment of the gut and the microbes that aid in food digestion would be different in each gut type. Many of our hormones, vitamins, and brain chemicals are made in the gut, so gut health can affect our mind, mood, and behavior, as well as the size and shape of our physical body. Many of the companies that test DNA now have programs to determine what kind of diet fits best with a specific genome.

Along with supplying the proper nutrients, the food we eat should nourish our soul and give us pleasure. This sends very important messages to our brain and increases chemicals, such as dopamine, that in turn will fuel fat burning and help us maintain a healthy weight. We can eat really healthfully, but if we perceive it as deprivation, it will not be as beneficial to us as if we enjoy our food and have our occasional treats as part of a well-balanced diet and lifestyle. Remember, it is our *perception* of our environment that sends signals to the cells of our body.

All of us, but particularly women in midlife, need to have increased amounts of antioxidants (found in brightly colored fruits and vegetables; vitamins A, C, and E) and a full spectrum of minerals, boron, and folic acid for healthy bones and adrenals. Even if we eat organically, our food has much lower mineral content these days, since modern agricultural practices do not allow the soil to rest and regenerate in the ways it used to in traditional farming practices. Minerals are very important in terms of adrenal and bone health.

It is also very important to make sure we get adequate amounts of the right kinds of fats. Omega-3 fatty acids improve the function of our nervous and immune systems, help our metabolism to work more efficiently, and decrease inflammation that can lead to heart disease. Also, keep in mind that cholesterol is the base from which all sex and stress hormones are made. It is my belief that the extremely low-fat diets that have been pushed on and embraced by women in the United States during the last couple of decades have added to the increase in hormone imbalance that I see every day in my practice.

Regardless of what kind of diet you prefer, your body needs high-quality protein, good fats, and carbohydrates to function effectively. You can get all of these micronutrients through healthy omnivore, vegetarian, or vegan diets. Ideally you should eat organically grown food whenever possible. Your diet should contain whole foods: brightly colored fruits and vegetables, complex carbohydrates, organic protein (which can be either plant or animal based), and healthy fats. For instance, breast cancer has been linked to some of the pesticides used on nonorganic fruits and vegetables and estrogen-like hormones used in raising livestock.

Not everyone can afford an organic diet, but there are certain foods that carry a heavier toxin load than others. You can do an internet search on "the Dirty Dozen" to find out which foods are highest in these toxins each year. Whenever possible, use organic dairy products, if you are going to eat dairy, since pesticides concentrate in breast milk. Most nutritionists agree, however, that adult humans have no need for dairy, and in terms of breast cancer risk, these foods carry the highest risk. Use hormone-free meats whenever possible, and wash fruits and vegetables before eating.

The fiber content of food is also very important. Research has shown that there is a 54 percent *decrease* in breast cancer risk with adequate fiber in the diet (30 grams of fiber per day is considered adequate for this). Plant foods and grains are the highest in fiber, and will also help you maintain a healthy weight. To help maintain a healthy weight, choose *nutrient-dense* foods (more nutrients per calorie) rather than foods that are high in fat and sugar. You will eat more if you eat empty calories, because your body is still looking for the nourishment it needs.

For healthy adrenals, it is important to maintain steady, normal blood sugar levels so that the adrenals do not have to tire themselves out, triggering fight-or-flight in order to constantly release sugar, fat, and protein into your system. If your blood sugar is not stable, and is spiking up and down, your body will store extra when it is high and trigger fight-or-flight to increase it when it is low, creating a vicious cycle and adding unwanted pounds.

If you are trying to heal your adrenals, have your largest meal in the morning, as this works with the natural rhythm of the adrenals, and make sure to eat protein within an hour of waking. Then eat something with protein, a good fat, and complex carbohydrate every three to four hours. These don't need to be huge meals—a handful of almonds is a good between-meal snack. Keeping your blood sugar stable assures your body that you are not in danger of starving and helps to switch it out of "store" mode. It also means that the adrenals do not have to work as hard to keep the blood sugar stable.

If you are not specifically trying to heal your adrenals, then follow whatever timing delivers steady energy and nourishment for your body. In fact, there is increasing evidence that intermittent fasting (eating within a window of ten hours in a day) helps the body to lose weight and maintain insulin sensitivity (the ability to clear sugar from the blood). Experiment and see what works best for you.

Stress

As we have seen in previous chapters, stress has far more to do with what ails us in modern life than people give it credit for. In fact, many of us don't realize how stressed we are. We have adapted to a level of stress that now feels normal to us. And remember, the body does not distinguish between good stress and bad stress. We might love what we are doing, but it has much the same effect on our body if we are doing too much of it.

So, we need to do what we can to lower the stress levels in our lives. Taking a close look at what nourishes us and brings us pleasure is a good place to start. (See the "good for me/bad for me" list on pages 51–52 for help with this.) Pleasure creates a positive feedback loop. When our body experiences pleasure, it releases hormones and other chemical messengers that tell our body it is safe, resulting in decreased stress levels and boosting our immune system. These messages have a ripple effect throughout the body. So we should aim to add more of what brings us pleasure wherever we can.

Next, we identify the things or people that drain us and don't give anything back and do our best to let go of these things. There are, of course, things that drain us that we are not able to let go of—family, for example, or a job that we are unable to change right away. In these cases, it is important to set new boundaries around these things.

So, the good stuff—more of it! Bring it on, and don't feel guilty! This is good self-care. Add more of what nourishes you and sustains you, and set new boundaries around the stressful things that you cannot change. Prioritize yourself and your healing. Twenty minutes of a practice that calms you—yoga, meditation, a walk, a bath, a power nap—once or twice a day can make a profound difference in your stress level by the end of the day. And each day that you conserve, you heal.

Exercise

Just as with nutritional information (and about everything else these days), information abounds as to what type and amount of exercise are optimal, and much of it is not in agreement. It is hard to know who or what to believe. There are studies that show that we need forty-five minutes of daily aerobic exercise to be healthy and studies that show five minutes of intense exercise twice a week is just as beneficial. It differs also as to whether we are training to build muscle mass, stamina, or just to maintain health. As with everything else, different things work better for different people. What is most important is choosing something that we will actually *do* and that fits into our schedule.

As with diet and gut type, there are even simple genetic tests that we can do to tell us if, from a genetic standpoint, our body would respond better to weight training or aerobic exercise in terms of maintaining a healthy weight. I am always leery of information that says that one way (their way) is right for everyone. This is usually connected to trying to sell us something, whether it be a perspective or a product! We have myriad differences as human beings, including different ethnic heritage, which has evolved from living under very different climates and conditions. We have different emotional histories and narratives that we have used to guide our lives. Why would we think that the same diet, exercise regimen, or lifestyle would be right for everyone? Yes, we are all human beings, but within that there is a great deal of variety.

Regular moderate activity does help to regulate weight, metabolism, and mood, and there is good evidence to show that it is preventive in terms of heart disease and breast cancer occurrence and reoccurrence. Find something you love to do and do it! This doesn't mean you need to take up a sport or a spin class if you don't enjoy that, but be active! Garden, go for a walk, dance! The sedentary lifestyle we currently live is not natural to the human body. It was only recently that we began to sit behind desks. Our ancestors did not have to go to aerobics class because they were doing physical labor as a natural part of their lives.

Research also shows that prolonged sitting is a risk factor for all causes of death, independent of how active we are physically. Sitting for extended periods raises the risk of developing type-2 diabetes and heart disease, as well as the risk of premature death. Risk for kidney disease goes up after three hours of sitting per day. So, it is worth taking a look at the rhythms of your life and seeing how much time is spent sitting (computer and TV are the biggest culprits, plus long commutes and lots of time spent in the car), and seeing if you can change that. Using a standing desk is a good strategy to help with this.

In the second half of life, and particularly while trying to heal the adrenals, exercise should be moderate, not overly strenuous. Strenuous aerobic exercise will make it more difficult for your adrenals to heal because it uses up energy that you need to conserve, more quickly. Studies also show that moderate exercise is actually more successful in burning fat, if this is a goal for you. Muscles can burn either fat or sugar. If you are exercising moderately but aerobically (with oxygen), you will burn fat. If your workout becomes too intense, your body can no longer supply enough oxygen to your muscles and it becomes anaerobic exercise. Then you are burning mostly sugar, which can actually slow your rate of fat loss.

Ideally, to burn fat, you want to be just below your maximum heart rate, which is determined by a formula based on age and current level of physical fitness. Walking is great, especially walking in nature, as is gentle bike riding or yoga. Weight-bearing exercise also helps to create strength, which in turn improves balance (making it less likely that you will fall), and builds strong bones.

Environment

A great deal of information has surfaced in the last two decades that indicates that many of the chemicals we come in contact with every day in the United States promote cancer growth in the body. Most European countries have banned these substances, along with genetically modified foods (GMOs), because the preponderance of evidence shows that they are harmful to human health. Our country will not ban them until there is "absolute proof," because they do not want to impinge on corporate rights to do business. Of course, many of the studies that would prove this unequivocally will never be done—the offending corporations themselves usually fund the studies, and it is not in their best interests to do so. Many corporations make money on both sides of the equation. They put the chemicals that cause cancer into the environment, they make the chemotherapy drugs with which we treat these cancers, and they are currently developing drugs to be used in "prevention" of cancers.

It is wise to be aware of the chemicals that can support cancer growth and that you are exposing yourself to on a regular basis through plastics, cleaning products, cosmetics, lotions, and pesticides. Go through your home and replace these with less toxic alternatives. Some examples:

- Avoid using chlorine bleach for laundry and household cleaning, or bleached products, such as coffee filters, paper napkins, toilet tissue, and tampons. The dioxin exposure from these products is significant, and regular use of these products can result in a lifetime exposure to this substance that exceeds acceptable levels. Hydrogen peroxide bleaches are a safe alternative for laundry; they break down into water and oxygen. You can buy unbleached sanitary products, if you are still having periods, or use a menstrual cup.

- Whenever possible, eat organic food or that which has not been raised with antibiotics and hormones.

- Drink water that does not contain chlorine and fluoride and avoid fluoride toothpaste. These substances compete with iodine at the level of receptors and negatively affect thyroid function.

- Reduce or eliminate the use of plastic products, particularly polyvinyl chloride (PVC). Many plastics leach hormone-disrupting chemicals into whatever they come in contact with, especially when heated. Never microwave in plastic containers or microwave food covered in plastic wrap! Always use glass or ceramic containers. The heat from the microwaves leaches chemicals from the plastic into your food.

- Avoid polybrominated diphenyl ethers (PBDEs), which are found in electronic equipment, furniture, and cars. These are found in the flame retardants used in fabrics, and in various plastics used in computer and car manufacturing. PBDEs contain hormone disruptors that are linked to reproductive damage and also negatively affect the thyroid. Whenever possible, choose clothing, carpet pads, bedding, and furniture upholstery made from natural fibers, such as wool, cotton, and hemp. Drive new cars with the windows open if at all possible, and give new products some time to off-gas in a well-ventilated area.

- Use wet cleaning rather than dry cleaning whenever possible for your clothes.

- Use personal care products that do not contain chemicals such as parabens and phthalates. Learn to read labels! The longer the ingredient list, the less likely you want to be putting it on your skin. Anything that goes onto your skin goes straight into your bloodstream and is ten times more potent to your body than if you swallowed it. There are wonderful oils that can be used on wet skin after a shower that are very effective moisturizers and actually nourish the skin.

- Do not use pesticides or herbicides on your lawn or in your garden. These contain xenoestrogens (chemicals that act like estrogen in the body and that bind with estrogen receptors). These are a known cancer risk. There are many safe alternatives to these compounds.

Sound daunting? It doesn't require completely changing your life in order to clean up your environment. Many of us use far more in the way of household cleaning products than is necessary. The marketing folks do a great job of making us think we need a different product for every task. We don't. Simply assess the number of products you use and how many chemicals each contains. Consolidating to a few effective, clean alternatives can make a huge difference in your exposure to these environmental toxins.

Getting Over the Hump

Lifestyle issues are some of the most difficult things for many women to shift. We know we ought to do it, we know the benefits—we *want* to, but we often find ourselves back at square one, feeling like a failure, like something is wrong with us. Why we engage in long-standing patterns that began when we were very young is sometimes the hardest thing to tease out, because we don't remember why they started in the first place.

There are many reasons why women might have difficulty sticking with changes they wish to make. For many, it is the larger rhythms of their lives that seem hard to shake. For example, someone might work at a job that requires her to get up very early and engage in a long commute. There isn't time to make breakfast. To make something the night before, when she is exhausted, seems equally impossible. So, the pattern continues.

Some may have physical limitations that they feel keep them from doing "what they know they are supposed to do," and they feel that it can only look one way (like having to go to the gym for it to count as exercise). That becomes the excuse that holds them back. If your work is sedentary, get up every half hour or so and move around. If your knees don't work, do more upper body activity. Do chair yoga, do laundry, walk to the mailbox! Everything counts.

Other women try to change everything at once; they make sweeping changes that are hard to sustain. There are some good books out there on changing habits, and most of them suggest that you start small, make it easy. If there *is* something you do reliably every day, try to connect the new behavior with the old one. (For instance, if you want to take supplements and can't remember to take them, pair it with brushing your teeth.) If possible, pair the new behavior to something pleasurable. If you can determine what your reward or "gain" is for a bad habit, maybe you can think of a better habit that gives you a similar gain, like choosing a relaxing bath instead of an hour of TV before bed, or dark chocolate instead of a bowl of ice cream. You would still get the relaxation and reward, but in ways that are better for your health. Whatever you feel you *can* do at a particular moment in time, do it—even if you can't do it reliably to begin with. I call this "moving toward the open space." Wherever you are, you are on the path.

Confusing "thinking" about something with "doing" it may also hold some of us back from implementing lifestyle changes. An example would be a woman who decides she is going to take up running again. She spends time researching what the best shoes are, and buys them. She reads about regimens, what burns the most fat, whether or not sprinting or power walking is the way to go. She buys new exercise clothes, she writes an exercise schedule in her calendar. She feels very busy engaging with her new habit. However, she *doesn't* get out there and run. The woman who just goes out for a relaxing walk, and does it a few times a week, is getting much farther down the path.

Often lifestyle adjustments are deal-breakers for women, when we begin to look at how we might improve our health. Making changes seems overwhelming. On some level, what we are currently doing works for us, even if the results are not what we might wish them to be. We feel caught in cycles of eating, lethargy, or stress that feel outside our power to change, so we feel overwhelmed and defeated even before we start. Consider, though, that the state of lethargy and the cravings for certain kinds of food might themselves be a product of lifestyle and its effects. They may have nothing to do with willpower or our ability to make changes in our lives.

For example, if your sleep has been disrupted for several months, you may have diminished levels of dopamine, which helps control the brain's reward and pleasure centers. Dopamine also helps regulate movement and emotional responses, and it enables us not only to see rewards but also to take action to move toward them. It significantly impacts our motivation. So, if your dopamine levels are low, your motivation to change or your capacity to feel reward or pleasure in your life will also be diminished, which will in turn make it harder to stick with something that doesn't feel like pleasure.

Many studies show that development of obesity is directly related to an increasing deficit in the brain's ability to sense rewards. A significant amount of the dopamine our body depends on is made in our gut. So, the lower your dopamine levels (either from sleep disruption or gut dysfunction due to diet or long-standing adrenal issues), the more likely you are to be obese and unable to break out of the cycle you are in.

Doing what it takes to bring good sleep back into the equation and eating foods that will increase levels of dopamine in the body can flip the switch that allows your brain to receive pleasure. Your motivation to be engaged will return and the pounds can fall away without flogging yourself to stick with a diet that *further* decreases dopamine because it feels like punishment, not reward. In the process, your adrenals will also begin to heal and your metabolism will stabilize. It is easy to do a search on which foods will increase various neurotransmitters in the brain.

So, once again, everything is connected. Sometimes making one small change will have a ripple effect that makes everything else easier and may take care of things further down the list without you lifting a finger. Take one step, any step that you can, and stick with it. You will see change.

Going Deeper

Looking at Your Lifestyle

So, let's begin with looking at lifestyle, with a bold eye, and tell ourselves the truth.

- How do you spend your days? Make a detailed list of the things you do in a day, even the little things such as picking up a teenager's clothes off of the floor.

- How many of these things are you doing for others? Are they capable of doing these things themselves?

- What tasks are for your own pleasure? Are they prioritized or do they fall off the list as soon as someone asks something from you?

- How well are the tasks of caring for the home (cooking, cleaning, shopping, laundry, driving) balanced between those who live there?

- Now, looking at your list above, make a "good for me/bad for me" list of your daily activities, as described in the previous section on stress. Be honest. What things in your life nourish you and bring you pleasure? How can you create more of those? What things are an energy drain and give nothing back? Let go of what you can. What things are a mixture of the two that you need to set boundaries around? How might you change things to decrease your stress, increase your pleasure, and create new boundaries around what you cannot let go of at this time?

- What are the rhythms in your life—the ones you choose and the underlying ones that move you through your day that you are hardly aware of? For those of us who work a job with regular hours, this will be part of the framework of our rhythm that is set from the outside. What does your internal tide tell you? Are your natural rhythms being honored in your life, as it stands? How, or why not?

- How is your sleep? If it is not good, what do you think is causing the disruption? Is it hot flashes? Blood sugar? Stress? Alcohol? Late bedtime? Do you have a bedtime ritual? What have you done to try to change this?

- What are you usually doing in the hour before bedtime?

- How many hours do you typically sleep? Is this all at one stretch or broken up? If broken, what wakes you up? Bladder? Hot flash? Hunger? Noise?

- What and what time of day do you tend to eat? Is there a pattern to it?

- How do your eating patterns change when you are stressed?

- What are you doing in addition to eating at each meal? Watching TV, reading, some other activity? Do you sit down for meals? Do you eat alone or with others?

- What kinds of foods do you typically crave? (Sugar is generally related to blood sugar, and salt is related to the adrenals.) Does this change for you at different times, and if so, what is involved in that? Do you eat protein throughout the day?

- What gut type would you imagine you have? Do you feel best when eating higher complex carbs? Higher protein? Higher fat? I am not asking what you eat to *lose the most weight* but rather what you are eating when you *feel* the best.

- What, if anything, keeps you from eating a healthy diet? Time? Stress? Finances? Emotions?

- Go through your cupboards and read labels. How much processed food is there? How much contains hidden sugars such as high fructose corn syrup?

- How much alcohol do you drink? Is it daily, weekly, or just when out with friends? How many drinks do you have at a time? How does this affect your sleep?

- Do you smoke cigarettes? Use marijuana or other substances or drugs? What do you go to them for? Relaxation? Pleasure? To "get away" from your life? How do they make you feel?

- How many hours a day do you sit, whether it is for reading, TV, computer work, driving, visiting with friends? How might you break that up so that you shorten the length of time at one sitting? How might you readjust things so that there is more activity and less sitting in your day (for example, maybe walk on a treadmill while you watch your TV show)?

- Can you think of a time in your life that your rhythms changed or your habits changed in a noticeable way (in a positive or negative direction)? What precipitated this? What changes did you notice to mood, energy, and overall health as a result of this?

- Are there any habits you wish to change? Is this easy or hard for you?

- Have you ever had success changing a habit? What made that possible?

- What do you have the greatest resistance to changing?

Looking at lifestyle and environmental issues can be intensely overwhelming, and changing them is often the deal-breaker for women when working toward better health. We often find this difficult because there is an emotional component to them and because these patterns begin so early in life. I would encourage you to be gentle and patient with yourself as you investigate this, and to remember that even small steps have a great ripple effect.

In this chapter, you have had an opportunity to look at your lifestyle with a bold eye, and you have likely found some things you would like to change. How you approach this will be very individual. Begin by thinking about your relationship to change—whether it excites you, scares you, makes you feel weary. The times you have been successful in changing a habit, how did that happen? Did you change everything all at once or make slow incremental changes? Look at things you want to change step by step, in terms of what would need to happen first in order to be successful. Remember, however, that thinking and strategizing about it are not the same as doing it.

It would also be helpful to shift your environment in such a way that would support these efforts. You might go through your kitchen and remove foods that are nonnutritive but represent a temptation. Being clear about all of the chemicals we are exposed to can be shocking. Go through your home and write down all of the cleaning products, lotions, cosmetics, shampoos, conditioners, laundry and dish detergents and softeners, and lawn care products that you come in contact with on a regular basis. Do you recognize the ingredients in these things? Give some thought to what you are exposing yourself to every day and where you might cut back in favor of some "cleaner" or more traditional items.

Once you have decided what you would like to shift, make a priority list. Take a look at what is most important and what might be easiest to shift first. Taking care of even one or two small, easier things makes space for bigger things and creates a track record of success for you. It might be something as simple as creating a rhythm for yourself or delegating household chores in a way that feels more equitable. Support is key here. Gather some allies before you begin.

Community

There are numerous people looking at the subject of longevity these days, not merely the fact of living longer, but living longer with the best quality of life. Most of these scientists approach this using the reductionist way of viewing medicine that we have in the West, cherry-picking data to focus on diet or exercise or certain micronutrients, looking to extract bioavailable substances to turn into supplements and find new ways to "cheat" death. However, there are several who are studying the people and cultures throughout the world who *are* long-lived, and looking at what they have in common. What they are finding may surprise you.

We can cherry-pick dietary data, or try to break down activity levels into calories burned, and in doing so, we would miss the most important aspects of what makes these cultures work in terms of longevity. We are so much more than our physical bodies, and we must look at ourselves as whole beings—physical, emotional, and spiritual—if we are going to have really useful information. All of that is encoded into our biology, and Nature's programming takes all of this into account.

When scientists looked at what variables were consistent across these long-lived cultures they studied, what they found was that a sense of purpose, social connections, and context had every bit as much—or more—to do with longevity as lifestyle components, such as diet and exercise, and the genetic makeup of the culture. From this study, called the *Blue Zones Project*, they were able to extrapolate that a sense of belonging was the base of the pyramid for vibrant long life (and this is particularly of interest to me in this digital age). Onto this base was added diet (largely composed of brightly colored whole plant foods, with strategies in place to avoid overeating), knowing one's purpose, and moving naturally (not numbers of minutes spent on a treadmill or at a gym, but gardening, walking, cooking, moving).

This was the formula for long and vibrant life, the keys to longevity: a sense of belonging, a sense of purpose, a reasonable diet, and a nonsedentary lifestyle.

It is important to remember that menopause is a juncture at which women make a decision to either move forward and engage with their lives in a creative way, or start to wind down. Think carefully about what you want to do—don't allow it to be an unconscious choice. It doesn't matter your age. It is never too late to start. Remember, you are already on the path. It is all connected. Just take a step and everything will line up to help you.

Going Deeper

Assessing Your Connections

Given that social connection, belonging, and purpose are so integral to living longer and having a fulfilling life, it is important to look at those things in our lives. Have you given conscious thought to this being a point of choice in your life? Do you feel this is in your control, or that you are trapped by circumstance? Many women feel trapped by jobs, debt, marriages, and commitments and feel that they cannot make the choices they need to make in order to live a more vibrant life. I would like for you to reconsider this, if you are one of those women. Even small changes or additions can have a significant ripple effect. So, think about the following things:

- Remember a time when you felt really good—vibrant and alive. What were you doing then? Who were you associating with? Where did you live? What specifically did it feel like? Where in your body? Stick with it until you can really remember it and feel it again in your body. This is important, as it builds a recent body memory.

- What or whom do you feel like you belong to? This could be in the form of people, a cause, a group that you engage with or trust. Who has your back? Who cares how you feel? Who *notices* when something is up?

- If you do feel this sense of belonging, what can you do to enhance that? If you don't, why do you think that is? Are you hesitant to trust? Are you too busy with taking care of others' needs? What might you do to take a step toward something that will nourish you in this way?

- When do you currently feel the most alive? What are you doing? What are you eating? Who are you hanging out with?

- What kind of exercise brings you *pleasure*? Not what brings the fastest "results," but what do you enjoy?

- Do you enjoy doing it alone or in company? Whose company?

- Do you have a strong sense of community support? If you were to be sick or injured, are there those you could call on who would happily help you out, and from whom you would feel comfortable accepting help?

- If you have identified what you enjoy and who you enjoy doing it with, what gets in your way? Are these excuses or true impediments?

- What are your favorite excuses? Do you believe them?

- What is one thing you can do, right now, to move toward what you want?

- Do you feel purpose in your life? If you do, and are not engaging with it, what gets in your way? If you do not, why do you think that is?

Community is one of the most important aspects of a vital elderhood. Elders who feel part of a community have better physical and emotional health. However, in our culture, many women come home to an empty house at the end of the workday. It is important to assess where our sense of connection comes from and whether there are people we can call on if we need physical or emotional support. This may come from family, activities, or friends.

Assess your support network and the groups you engage with that bring you joy and a sense of purpose. How can you make more of this in a way that you can continue to engage with as you age? Think about beginning something that made you feel alive when you were younger, that you have let lapse because of work or other obligations. Take a class that you have been putting off. You might also find a meetup group in your area—a community with similar interests—or form one of your own, such as a book group or dinner club.

PART TWO

Sexuality and Relationship

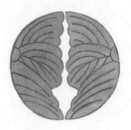

Chapter 7

The Continuum, Continued . . .

If anything is sacred, the human body is sacred. —Walt Whitman

In the same way that the concept of the continuum allows us to understand and connect our earliest experiences to our hormone balance as adults and the way our bodies move into menopause, we can also see that there is a significant connection between our early experiences and the development of our sexuality and its expression during all phases of our lives. For many women, both their experience and expression of sexuality change during menopause. This will be explored in detail in later chapters of the book, but it is helpful to place this in the context of all the years that have come before.

Scientists who study the brain tell us that we spend the first six years or so of our life in a mild version of a hypnotic trance, with our brain acting essentially as a tape recorder, downloading information and experiences without the benefit of any significant analysis to filter those experiences. What we receive, we essentially receive without question, as truth. Because of this, what we experience and receive in our infant years—that is, our preverbal years—literally lives in every cell of our body. This is how it is possible to come to adulthood, having processed the traumas and distorted messages from our early years, have insight about them and do any amount of therapy, yet still be ruled by them, no matter how subtly. We act as if they are true, because on the level of our body and our "deep knowing," they are. It doesn't matter so much what the mind knows; it is what the body remembers.

As infants, we are exquisitely sensitive to sound, light, touch, and taste, and we're very highly attuned to our emotional environment. An infant's whole body and being is essentially one big sponge, soaking up experience, acclimating and attuning itself to the environment it has been born into. This is epigenetics in action; this is survival.

The way our mother or caregiver handled our infant body and connected with us emotionally has everything to do with our ability as a child, budding adolescent, and young adult to trust our body, feel comfortable in it, receive touch openly, and feel ourselves worthy of love. Whether our mother or caregiver touched our infant body with gentleness, confidence, permission, and warning, especially when changing diapers, can set the stage in an unconscious, every-cell-of-our-body way for how safe we feel and how we respond to sexual contact later in life.

A caregiver who changes diapers abruptly, efficiently, and less than gently; who uses rough or cold wipes, which can be shocking to an infant's sensitive skin; and who makes no emotional connection to the infant while doing this, can create a context where on some level the infant feels it needs to distance itself from this touch. The infant is therefore somewhat shut down to it. Also, if the caregiver reacts to the infant's bodily wastes with disgust and avoidance, whether or not anything is said out loud, that message is transmitted as well, and the infant adjusts its self-concept to include that response.

However, it also seems to be true that the intent or quality of an emotion or connection carries more weight in the end than the actual way our body is handled. Studies carried out in orphanages have shown that a baby can be efficiently cared for and yet not have the emotional connection that comes from a loving caregiver and be far more damaged than the child whose caregiver is inept or inexperienced, but who connects to the child emotionally and with love.

I remember when entering a new hospital as a midwife, nurses would be completely thrown by the fact that I would speak to the newborns while examining them, telling them ahead of time that I was going to put a cold stethoscope on their chest, wipe their face, turn them over, give them an injection, or put a tube down their throat. I would touch them gently, look into their eyes when I was talking with them, and wait until I felt the relaxation under my hand telling me that they were ready before proceeding.

In the beginning, there was some inevitable eye-rolling in response to this. However, over time, when the nurses saw the infants' responses and that exams and procedures could be carried out with quiet, cooperative babies instead of being fought every inch of the way, they were entranced. Without fail, a couple of months down the road, many more nurses were engaging in this behavior and reaping the benefits of two-way communication. Babies are incredibly sensitive, sentient beings.

Though there has been some shift in recent years, for decades we were taught in medicine that newborns cannot feel, understand, or remember pain; they are just "baby meat." Anyone who is paying attention around newborns knows that this couldn't be further from the truth—babies communicate quite well—but the textbooks, until very recently, had staunchly maintained this to be true. Circumcision continues to be performed largely without anesthesia, in the belief that the infant brain is not developed enough to remember pain. And any mother who thinks she sees a smile is just deluded; it is only gas.

So, although we sometimes think of our sexuality as something that begins to develop at puberty, who we are sexually is created from our very first days on earth, even in the womb. For instance, several studies show that the physical makeup and response of the brains of gay men and lesbian women differ from their heterosexual counterparts and more closely resemble the brains of the opposite-sexed heterosexual. You might say, then, that our first experiences, those experiences that will begin to shape who we will become as a sexual being, begin even before birth, as our brains form.

We really cannot separate our sexuality from the rest of who we are. Our brain is wired to our mother's hormone balance in the womb, and this sets the stage. Our early experiences of touch as an infant, our family's attitudes toward bodies and nudity, and our parents' responses to us when we explored our body all create early context. As we then move out into the world, the media adds its two cents to the messages of our family and their ideas about what girls should and should not do or wear, or how girls should act; whether we should be allowed to take physical risks or must be more demure than boys, regardless of our innate proclivities or desires. Religious training also plays a huge role for many girls. All of these influences already inform who we find ourselves to be when we begin to think of ourselves for the first time as a sexual being, and they also color what our expectations might be as to how we will be received in this regard.

Unfortunately, many girls are sexualized at an early age, against their will, through inappropriate sexual contact or exposure to sexual contexts. Studies show that depending on whether there was force, penetration, or involvement of a trusted family member, these experiences can have the effect of either over-sexualizing girls (having earlier onset of menarche, earlier sexual experience, and teen pregnancy) or creating sexual aversion, depression, self-mutilation, revictimization, trust issues, or cognitive impairment.

In addition to the psychological and emotional symptoms, many stress-related physical symptoms occur, such as obesity, hormone imbalances, and adrenal fatigue—all signs of severe stress.

By the time a girl reaches puberty, she has already soaked up many influences. While the context and values of her family are initially the strongest influence, the media culture begins to pull ahead at puberty, since we are now marinated in it from a very early age. Her peer group also has a very strong influence in this regard.

Going Deeper

What Your Body Knows

Knowing your personal history regarding your sexual development, how you inhabit your body and respond to touch, can help to increase your awareness and understanding of where you *currently* find yourself in regard to these things. Knowing this allows you to be more compassionate and accepting of where you find yourself now, and is invaluable when trying to create change.

If you have awareness or strong suspicion that you might have been sexually abused in your early years, you might want to ensure that you have a therapist or support system in place before delving deeply into some of these self-inquiry questions.

We touched on some of these themes in earlier sections of self-inquiry, but let's look at them in more detail, and in the context of what we have just been exploring. Sometimes looking at the same thing from a slightly different angle will bring out new information.

- What do you know about your newborn days? Were you nursed? Were you held a lot or kept in a playpen or chair? Were you the firstborn or did your parents have experience by the time you arrived?

- What was the attitude about bodies in your home growing up? Was there a relaxed attitude and comfort with nudity, touching, physical contact? Or not?

- How comfortable were you in exploring the boundaries of your physicality, taking risks and trying new things? Was this exploration encouraged or discouraged in your family? For what reasons?

- What was your relationship with your body as child? Did you trust it? Feel healthy? Or were you taught to worry about every little symptom or scraped knee? What or who influenced your relationship to your body?

- When did you become aware of the differences between boys' and girls' bodies? How did this come about? Are there particular memories that go along with this?

- What was the response of your parents if they caught you playing "doctor" or engaging in exploration of your body with other children?

- Were your parents glad you were a girl? Did you feel your parents had specific expectations or visions for you because you were a girl? If so, how did that express itself?

- Did *you* grow up being happy you were a girl?

- As you hit puberty, what were your mother's and father's messages to you about your body? About your sexuality? Did they see this as a natural unfolding and support you through your early explorations with dating or attraction, or did they give off messages of fear or that your sexuality was somehow wrong? How did they show this?

- What was your mother's relationship to her own body and sexuality as yours was beginning to express? Did your mother support you? Compete with you? How did this show itself?

- What role did religion play in your home? What did your religion teach you about what was right or what was wrong in terms of becoming a woman and forming relationships with potential partners?

- Think about any experiences that might have felt "wrong" to you as a child. Are there any that you now might question in terms of their appropriateness? What was the story you told yourself (or were told, if you shared them) about these experiences?

- Were you sexually abused as a child? If so, what steps have you taken to heal from that trauma? If you haven't sought treatment or help from a support system, what holds you back?

How we relate to our bodies as women and sexual beings is not only very personal but also an area in which most women are particularly vulnerable. Perhaps looking at this from the perspective of a continuum has helped you to understand something new about the way you inhabit your body and the way your sexuality developed. If there is new material to uncover or understand here, have a conversation with your mother or those in your family who might help you connect the dots with any early material you feel is relevant to the way you inhabit your body now. If you are able, and you think it would be helpful, you might contact early partners.

If you are interested in knowing more about what babies actually know and experience, connect with the Association for Prenatal and Perinatal Psychology and Health. You may be surprised! The information is fascinating. Remember, babies aren't just babies. They're us!

Chapter 8

Becoming a Lover

Lovers don't finally meet somewhere.
They're in each other all along. —**Rumi**

O ur first experiences with potential lovers often play a critical role in cementing how we feel about ourselves as women. Depending on whether we felt seen, safe, and attractive, these experiences can deeply color whether we feel we will be seen and loved in our ongoing sexual lives. It is unfortunate that such formative experiences often happen when our brains are still so much in flux, our emotions so volatile, and our ability to "read" situations at an all-time low.

Our hormones are also in flux during menopause, and sometimes when everything seems to be changing at once, these issues pop back up for us, even if they have been gone for years. We are once again uncertain about what we are becoming. It is useful to explore what it was like the first time around, in order to be ready for what might surface during the menopausal years.

The Yin and the Yang

Spiritual traditions for thousands of years have been aware of the dual nature of our universe, and each tradition speaks of it in its own language—the light and the dark, the yin and the yang, the above and below, the tantric inbreath and outbreath of the Universe. Nothing is static; everything moves, everything cycles.

We move toward, we move apart. It is why Nature polarizes us so strongly, through our hormones, during the reproductive years. We must have "apartness," otherness, in order to come together once more.

Our culture ascribes different characteristics to maleness and femaleness. We also ascribe maleness and femaleness to certain hormones—estrogens being considered female and androgens being considered male. But, in fact, we each contain the All; we are each a universe unto ourselves. However, during the reproductive years, we tend to hang out on one end of the pole more than the other because of the way hormones inform our bodies and brains. We are in a less integrated state than we are in either our "latent," or post-reproductive, years.

Characteristics attributed to maleness are generally active or assertive. Maleness is seen as the realm of the manifest, the seen, having to do with light or fire, penetration, the chase, the hunt, dominance. Genitally, it is very focused and goal-oriented. When out of balance, this leads to aggression and violence. Female qualities are perceived as those that are unseen—the seed, the receptive, gentleness, the sensate, and the submissive. The female is the Mystery, or the dark, loamy place that receives the seed, nurtures it to fruition, and sends it back out into the world. When out of balance, this expresses as the victim or the doormat.

It is important to remember, however, that as humans, we are not either/or. Some women embody a more yang energy and some men embody more yin. We are a unique combination of the two, depending on our innate qualities and cultural influences. When looking at the yin-yang symbol from ancient Taoism, it is clear that each principle has within it the seed of the other; it is a continuum to be moved along, to bring forth what is needed at any given time, in the fluid dance that is the whole.

The Flower to the Bee

Attraction, that magnetic pull to another, is a many-layered thing. Smell, hearing, and visual cues are all involved, as well as hormones and pheromones (chemical factors secreted by the body that trigger social responses in members of the same species). The sequence of events, or dance, that occurs during attraction and flirtation appears to be the same in humans across cultures. Perhaps it is not surprising that many of the hormones involved in initial attraction are the same as those in the fight-or-flight response, since at root we're deciding to approach or flee.

If approach is the decision, then there is a particular sequence of events that unfolds in terms of body language. First, a person will make exaggerated movements to call attention to themselves. Then, if things progress and the couple is more comfortable with each other, they begin to mirror each other's movements. This is actually a basic form of attachment or bonding that we also see between mothers and their newborns. A new baby will synchronize its movements to the sound of its mother's voice. This is called entrainment.

Meanwhile, the potential partner has to "smell right" for things to progress. This is where pheromones come in. Pheromones are made in the apocrine (sweat) glands, located in armpits, around the nipples, and in the groins of both males and females, but these chemicals differ from sweat. These chemicals are a major part of the attraction dance. Male pheromones play a role not only in attraction but also in regulating the menstrual cycles of women, inducing ovulation, and even letting the body know on a chemical level whether a potential mate has a complementary immune system and is therefore genetically a good match.

Not only does the particular "smell" of someone matter but studies have found that what attracts us at different phases of our menstrual cycle is very different. During ovulation, women tend to be drawn to men with more classic masculine qualities, such as greater facial symmetry, a deeper voice, more muscle tone, and dominant behaviors. From Nature's perspective, these men are considered to be more fertile and have better genes to offer to a potential child.

At other times of the menstrual cycle, women might choose very different qualities, such as intelligence, emotional availability, and the ability to be a good provider.

What I find very interesting is that studies have also found that these pheromone-driven behaviors no longer hold true in women using birth control pills or hormonal contraceptives. The contraceptives appear to disrupt some of the chemical signals that affect a woman's attractiveness to men and a woman's own preferences for romantic partners. This makes total sense in that hormonal forms of contraception prevent ovulation and disrupt the "cycle" of the menstrual cycle. These contraceptives make things steady-state throughout the month, thereby tricking the body into thinking it is already pregnant and suppressing ovulation.

Since there is no cycle, the cyclic preferences get wiped out as well. Women using hormonal forms of contraception no longer experience greater desire for a more masculine partner at ovulation (because they don't ovulate), nor are they able to distinguish any longer those partners with a different immune system from theirs. Likewise, men no longer show shifting interest in women based on where they are in their cycle, because those cues are no longer present. I have often wondered if the prevalence of hormonal contraception and the way it disrupts Nature's attraction dance has anything to do with the rising divorce rate or people feeling that they have somehow ended up with the wrong partner.

Love or Lust?

There are several stages that we go through as we fall in love and then form attachments and long-lasting relationships, and most of them are hormonally driven. Given that our hormones go through major change at menopause, some women wake up and look at their partner and think, *How did I get here?* It is useful (and I think fascinating) to see what brings us together in the first place, and remembering "how we got here" sometimes helps to bring us back. It is also useful to note that just as hormones drive these various states of attraction, our changing hormone levels at midlife may leave us feeling differently about our partners or what we find ourselves attracted to than we did before menopause.

Lust is considered the first stage of love, and is driven mainly by the hormones estrogen and testosterone. Several significant studies have shown that regardless of gender or sexual orientation, age ten is the mean age of first sexual attraction. However, a person is not ready to play out this attraction until levels of estrogen and testosterone are sufficient to cause puberty and the biological capability for reproduction.

Surprised that your ten-year-old is dreaming of movie stars? Maybe you shouldn't be. Films and literature alike are filled with examples of young crushes, and you may even remember your own. It might have been on a boy, or a girl, or your teacher, or a movie star. This ramping up of attraction and sexual awareness all has to do with the adrenal glands, which reach maturation around age ten.

Both male and female infants are born with adult levels of sex hormones and maintain these during the first days of their lives. This makes sense in that the infant in the womb has been hooked up directly to the mother's bloodstream, which is circulating very high levels of sex hormones during pregnancy. After a few months, the sex hormones fall to a very low level and then remain low (hence our relative androgyny during our early years) until the adrenal glands, ovaries, and testes mature and begin to create adult sexual characteristics and eventually the ability to reproduce.

The adrenal glands, being the second greatest source of our sex hormones next to the ovaries and testes, kick-start this process around age ten, pumping new levels of DHEA and other adrenal hormones into the system, which then turn into estrogen, testosterone, and progesterone. Neurotransmitters (brain chemicals) play a huge role in attraction as well. If we are low in certain neurotransmitters, it can have a significant effect on our libido, our motivation to seek out a sexual partner, and our capacity to experience pleasure.

In the early stages of attraction, when we are first falling in love and can't think of anything else but the object of our affection, levels of adrenaline and cortisol are increased in the bloodstream. Remember, these are the hormones that are high during fight-or-flight, and "approach or flee" is one of the earliest moves in the flirtation dance, so this makes a lot of sense. Adrenaline is the reason that our heart races, we begin to sweat a little, or we become a bit tongue-tied when we are in the presence of our new love.

Our levels of the neurotransmitter dopamine also surge in the early stages of attraction. This chemical is an integral part of the desire-and-reward loop and has a lot to do with motivation and movement. This higher level of dopamine is why new couples often feel increased energy, less need for sleep or food, and a sense of very focused attention on and pleasure from the smallest details having to do with our Beloved. Our energy, self-confidence, and focus will be much higher when levels of this neurotransmitter are optimal.

Serotonin is another one of love's most important chemicals. It recharges our brain and has a lot to do with mood and appetite. (Low serotonin leads to depressed mood and food cravings, mostly for salty things.) Serotonin is one of the reasons we can't stop thinking about our Beloved. An Italian study of couples who had been "madly in love" for less than six months showed the same high levels of circulating serotonin as someone with obsessive-compulsive disorder.

It should be no surprise the hormones that mediate attachment and attraction as adults also mediate our very first attachments, that of babies to their mothers. In fact, it would be true to say that mothers and babies fall in love with each other in the same way (hormonally) that adults do.

During orgasm and childbirth alike, there is a surge of the hormone oxytocin, the love hormone, a very powerful hormone that creates deep feelings of attachment. Oxytocin also creates connections between couples who make love—the more often they make love, the deeper the connection. It is what causes bonding between mothers and babies. Oxytocin causes breasts to automatically release milk when a mother hears her baby cry. Take oxytocin away and animal mothers will reject their young. Give oxytocin to female animals who have never had sex and they will begin to care for another female's young, protecting them as if they were their own.

Sounds great, right? *Where can I get some? Is there a pill I can take?* Unfortunately, oxytocin, being a peptide hormone, can only go in one direction—from brain to bloodstream—in order to create this effect. You cannot take it and have it travel to the brain to cause these feel-good feelings.

Going Deeper

Your Love Stories

In this section, take particular note of whether you feel body sensations when you think about these early experiences. For example, if you had an experience of rejection, where did you feel it in your body? What did it feel like? Was this in response to a particular comment or action?

Here are some questions to ask yourself to begin to look at the kind of partners and relationships you are attracted to.

- What were your earliest memories of girls and boys being different in more than just a physical way?

- What characteristics did you attribute to being male or female? What were you told about each gender's attributes? How did your own sense of gender align with or deviate from what you were told?

- Were you a traditionally feminine girl or a tomboy? In what ways did you express this?

- At what age did you experience your first crush? Who was the object of your desire? A friend? A teacher? A public figure? Were they male or female?

- How did it feel to have this first crush? Did you feel you could tell anyone about it? Did you feel these feelings would be accepted or ridiculed?

- Did you tell your first crush about your feelings, if it was someone you knew?

- When do you first remember feeling sexual sensations in your body? What did you think was happening?

- What about your first experiences with attraction? Were you accepted? Rejected? How did you express your attraction? Did the object of your desire even know?

- What kind of men or women did you find yourself being attracted to? At age ten? Age thirteen? Age sixteen? Adult years? Has this changed at midlife?

- How do you know you are attracted to someone? What specifically do you feel?

- Were you ever attracted to someone you "shouldn't" have been? Who decided they were inappropriate? What about this person resonated with you?

- Is this still consistent today or has it changed? If changed, in what ways?

- As you got older, was there a "type" that you were attracted to? What were the characteristics of this person?

- What experiences (or books or movies) went into forming this template?

- In your relationships to date, how long does the intense initial attraction usually last? What are the typical reasons your attraction wanes?

- If the attraction fades, what do you tend to do? Leave the relationship? Talk about it and try to recapture a closer intimacy? Just live with it?

- Have you experienced the loss of attraction that later returned in a relationship? If so, what helped to bring it back?

As you look at your path toward who you have become today as a lover, what phases your attractions passed through, and who you are *now* in relationship to yourself and someone else, a lot of feelings may arise. Some of the information that you uncovered and what went into your template of attraction might be surprising. Did you find you were attracted to the people with whom you would really be most compatible? Or were you acting out of some past pattern that you were familiar with or a cultural expectation that didn't represent what you truly hoped to create with someone? Knowing this can help you create a more realistic picture of what a compatible partnership looks like for you now.

Take a look at your current attractions. See if you can determine at what age your template was formed. Is it still appropriate for you now? If not, take some time to feel into what would be appropriate for you at this stage of life.

In the same way that you had a path that brought you here, your partner—if you are with one—did as well. Ask your partner about their early templates and how they have changed. Do those templates still serve them? Share your stories and what you see as being important *now* and in the future. See if you can look at the future together and create something that serves you both.

You might question whether you ended up with the right person. If you feel you did not, see if you can figure out where you got off track and what you can do right now to move toward more authenticity.

Chapter 9

How Our Relationships Form

When we're incomplete, we're always searching for
somebody to complete us. When, after a few years or
a few months of a relationship we find that we're still
unfulfilled, we blame our partners and take up with
somebody more promising. This can go on and on—series
polygamy—until we admit that while a partner can
add sweet dimensions to our lives, we, each of us, are
responsible for our own fulfillment.   —Tom Robbins

The menopausal years are a time when many relationships
fail or go through major changes. Part of this is due to
shifts in estrogen from *estradiol* (Nature's baby-making
hormone) to *estriol* (the estrogen that stimulates the creative centers
in our brain). This shift often makes women less likely to put aside
their own needs, wants, and desires for those of other people.
We get back on our own lists, so to speak. We may reevaluate
everything about our life, and sometimes our partner is not able
to be flexible with the directions we want to take. Sometimes we
have just become so used to each other's presence that we no longer
"see" each other.

Relationships generally go through three stages. First, there is
the infatuation stage, where we are struck by the lightning bolt

of our Beloved. Everything they do or say is precious to us. The hormones of love are flowing strongly and this holds us together through all of the things that will later drive us crazy.

The brain is not able to sustain this level of stimulation forever, so the hormones and the intense feelings eventually begin to fade, and we come to a place of neutrality. Science tells us that this happens anywhere from two to three years into a relationship. When we're able to look at our partner neutrally, we also begin to see them more realistically. During this second phase, we often begin to try to change our partner. We want them to be the way we want them, so that we can continue to feel about them the way we did in the beginning. We want that high back. It was all so great when they were "perfect" or we found their imperfections adorable.

People do not change easily, however—and most, not at all. We want to be who we are, sometimes quite stubbornly so. We dig in our heels. No one is going to change us. This is often the phase in which infidelities occur. We want that rush again. Men are generally looking for sexual validation. Women are generally looking for the feelings of deep connection they had and now feel they have lost.

If a couple survives this second phase, it moves on to phase three, where we are seeing our partner clearly and realize we are not going to change them—what we see is what we get. Many couples divorce at this point, usually about four or five years into the marriage, or they try to stay together "for the sake of the children." If the couple can move through this phase, however, each seeing and accepting the other for the very real human being they each are, then the chances are good that this can be a growthful and productive long-term relationship. Couples that move beyond this second phase are usually able to see the pros and cons of their partner's personality and ways of being in the world, and how those traits complement their own. They move into a rhythm that respects both but allows for difference and space in the relationship. And the hormonal tidal wave will sweep through again from time to time; it is not gone for good.

There are a few things I find interesting in terms of what we know drives love and attachment. First of all, with the amount of hormonal contraception being used, we are not as likely to be choosing the same partners that we would in a natural world. We are hooking up with and marrying men that we are not necessarily biologically compatible with. When the tidal wave of bliss recedes, we are often left standing on the beach wondering how we got here with this person. *What were we thinking?*

Second, Nature is largely playing matchmaker, and while we think we are consciously choosing, our neurotransmitters are choosing for us. Our brains imprint to early sexual experiences, both what we encounter in books and films or on television and what we actually experience as babies, children, and teenagers. These experiences create a template in our brains, and we often move toward people who fit a certain mold but are not the ones we would truly be compatible with.

Third, especially in this country, girls are brought up on the fairy tale: the meet-cute, the love dropping out of the sky, the Prince Charming with few flaws (and if they have flaws, they are adorable and are always overcome by the heroine). I think it is significant, though, that these stories always end at the wedding and conclude "and they lived happily ever after." We believe it because they say so, but we never get a look into the actual years after the marriage to see what comes next. What does it take to live happily ever after? We only have half the story before our fantasies are created and we embark on our own adventures.

These stages also apply to same-sex couples. Sexual orientation is a continuum that people fall along as well. While some people may be hardwired for same-sex love, others may be bisexual, pansexual, asexual, or find themselves with different attractions at different times of their lives. We are influenced by our brain's development, as well as early experiences, levels of safety, and hormonal factors. Our potential as human beings is rich and varied and very rarely as black and white as we have been taught.

Going Deeper

Looking at Your Relationships

Here are some questions to help you dive into looking at how your ideas and desires around relationship formed. I would encourage you to consider working with the ones you are not drawn to as well as the ones you are. Sometimes we avoid what we don't want to look at, and there is a lot of rich information packed in there. Looking back through your life, consider:

- Did you grow up in a household with one parent or two? If one, how did that affect the parent that remained?

- Was there grief in one parent from the loss of a spouse through death?

- If one parent left the other, was there resentment toward that person or the entire sex of the person who left? If so, how were these attitudes transmitted to you? How did that parent get their needs for adult companionship met?

- If there were two parents in your household, what was their relationship like? Was there a sense of ease between them? Did they seem to respect each other? Did they appear to divide duties along gender roles (regardless of whether it was a heterosexual or homosexual couple)? Were they openly affectionate?

- When you were young, what were your friendships with the opposite sex like? How did that change once you started dating?

- Is there a particular book, movie, or "mantra" from your parents or family that defined for you what a *good* relationship was or "the way you would want it to be" for you? (Go as far back as you can to see what the early images were. Remember that Disney played a huge role in this for women now in their sixties and seventies.) What was that myth?

- Did that myth have more to do with the emotional feeling tone of the relationship? The physical aspect? The status or trappings?

- Once you began to engage in relationships of your own, what were your experiences? How did they compare to the myth you were brought up on?

- How old were you when you had your first boyfriend or girlfriend? What drew you to them?

- Was your first relationship one of deep connection? Were you able to be vulnerable with each other? Or was it more to just have a boyfriend or girlfriend and fit in or look good?

- What kinds of things did you do together? How did you express or hide your true self with this person?

- When did you have your first sexual relationship? Was it respectful? Consensual? Did you feel seen? How long did it last? How did it end?

- Did your adult relationships closely resemble your parents' relationship in any way? Did they have similar dynamics, issues, or problems to what you saw your caregivers experiencing?

- Is there a particular phase in a relationship that you find yourself having trouble with? Have you successfully moved past these phases? What did you do that worked? That didn't work?

- Is there a point in a relationship in which you often stop and cannot move forward? Why do you feel this is?

Quite often, it comes as a surprise when we see how much of our attitudes toward the opposite sex come from the environment we marinated in growing up. These attitudes are often not even spoken of, as such. They're just presented as the way things are, so we don't question them, and sometimes we don't even realize we hold them. As you spend time looking back over the events that formed your viewpoint on relationships (and helped to create the expectations you have of someone else and what is possible), try to be very present with these memories. Notice whether you have feelings in any particular part of your body when you think about these experiences. If you focus on those feelings, notice where in your body they reside. Notice their qualities. If they are not positive feelings, allow yourself to explore them nevertheless, and try not to distance yourself from them. Notice whether there are other experiences you can connect to those same feelings in your body. What further comes up if you are able to do this? Making these connections can help us to better understand what the emotions and qualities were that formed our beliefs of what is possible for us, even if we don't remember specifics.

Talk with your partner about *their* early attractions and relationships. Identify what went into forming *their* expectations and sense of what is possible. See how those relate to yours. Notice whether there are fundamental differences at this point in time. Look at where both of you stand in relationship to earlier ways of being. Look at what might be possible going forward if you chart a course together.

Chapter 10

Sex and Culture

If our sex life were determined by our first
youthful experiments, most of the world
would be doomed to celibacy. —P. D. James

Menopause is a time when women often begin to explore
what is truly authentic for them in their sexuality. Everything is changing—our hormonal balance
changes and our reproductive urge diminishes. In order to know
what is authentic for us, it is important to explore the early influences in our lives that pointed us in a certain direction.

As mentioned in earlier chapters, we are incredibly sensual, responsive organisms finely tuned for survival. Our body
is made to feel, sense, and receive information. Our brain is
designed to make sense of that information and detect patterns.
Our behavioral responses are based on that information. This is
how we survive.

The quality of touch we receive early in life and the responses
of our caregivers to our exploration of our body and the world
around us all inform our brain and the template it is creating about
who we are and what we can expect from the world. Babies are
programmed to explore their world with abandon, yet many parents and caregivers—sometimes out of their own upbringing, and
especially if they are inexperienced or overwhelmed—constantly
restrict and try to contain this exploration.

If a child is always told no or that they are bad when they step outside of bounds or explore their own body, then this sets up deep patterns in the brain. Remember, our experiences prior to about age six are received without question, as truth. In many families where there is a strong religious overlay, a girl may grow up feeling that any exploration of her body is shameful or that she is wicked, immoral, and not worthy of love. We carry these feelings into later stages of our lives. Many women who are now in their sixties or older experienced a fair amount of shame in their upbringing.

Not only does this early shaming strongly inform a woman's self-concept, but it also biases her toward self-observation later on when she becomes sexual. Because she is essentially split on the issue—her young programming tells her she is bad, even if she no longer believes that to be true—a part of her is outside, watching when she engages in sexual activities, and she cannot be fully present, which inhibits her ability to be sexually open and fully orgasmic.

The media's promulgation of a very narrow and specific body type associated with attractiveness also has women self-observing a lot during sex. Only about 3 percent of women look like the media ideal. The rest of us often find it difficult to "get naked," as it were, with full abandon. Many women have told me that they spend almost the whole time they are making love wondering how they look to their partner, or making sure they position themselves in such a way that they will look thinner or what they consider to be more attractive. They are unable to be fully present and abandon themselves to the experience of sex because of their level of self-observation.

We are doing better at teaching the basic anatomy and physiology of reproduction than we used to. However, in our current culture, where sex is used to sell everything from lawn mowers to toothpaste, most of us still arrive at our first love relationship and first sexual experiences knowing very little about how our body works in terms of arousal and response, or what to expect in terms of anything other than basic mechanics. Relatively little is taught, except in the movies, about our sexuality in relationship to another human being, other than being told by school and church to "Just say no," which isn't very useful in the face of a body awash in hormones telling us to do just the opposite.

In our schools, we barely teach anything about prevention of pregnancy and nothing at all about human sexual response and creation of relationships. This is likely out of a fear that it will be seen as encouraging teen sex, or sex before marriage, and the assumption that such education is the purview of parents. It should be, but by and large, parents are either ill-equipped or unwilling to talk to their children about relational aspects of sexuality, and our adolescents are left to flounder.

Truth be told, many adults are floundering, too. In my gynecology practice, I frequently encountered women who did not know during what time of their cycle they were fertile, how pain during intercourse could be avoided by allowing for full arousal, or what sort of stimulation was most likely to lead them to orgasm. Both they and their partners had come to adulthood and through many years of sexual experience without being provided this information.

This means that our teens and young people are largely ignorant about how the body works sexually as they begin their relationships, or they are learning from other misinformed teenagers or, worse yet, Hollywood, whose portrayals of sex are, for the most part, highly unrealistic. Sex scenes in the movies are generally either over-romanticized or overcharged, and very male in their perspective; everyone gets there fast, because this is what sells, and you only have a few minutes of screen time that you can devote to a sex scene. This is a problem, especially given the fact that our early experiences set the template for our sexual self-concept, our later sexual experiences, and what we find ourselves drawn to over and over again.

Our earliest impressions are critical, because of the way our perceptions inform our physical reality. In my practice over the years, I have seen time and time again where women feel that they are inadequate or abnormal sexually because they are not constantly turned on or don't have exaggerated, multiple orgasms and their lovemaking does not look like it does in the movies. They think that what they are seeing in the media is normal, what they should be, and this misconception is reinforced by the fact that most people don't speak openly about their own sexuality or sexual practices, especially if they feel they are somehow wanting. Therefore, women have nothing to compare their own experiences to. Often teenage boys or immature lovers will play on this, making a woman feel that something is wrong with her, because the lover thinks it should look a different way, or their own sexual self-esteem is shaky. These women and men have had no opportunity to find out who they are authentically, in terms of their sexuality.

The way the brain is structured to receive stimulation also plays its part. A man's brain and a woman's brain are wired differently in terms of desire and sexual arousal. This makes total sense from an evolutionary perspective. Men are wired to be visually stimulated and easily aroused, as it assists in widely spreading their seed. For women, the sense of connection and safety are paramount before they can be fully aroused. (Though, of course, we also enjoy looking!)

The media's portrayal of constantly aroused women and overly romanticized men often leads to unrealistic expectations in our relationships as well. Men expect women to have libidos that look like theirs, and women feel this pressure and feel as if they are not whole women if they do not. Likewise, women often yearn for or expect their guys to be like them—romantic, dreamy-eyed, and focused on connection. They feel disappointed, angry, and often unloved because their man doesn't want to spend the amount of time they do talking, cuddling, hand-holding, and gazing into each other's eyes. This can lead to great misunderstandings about whether someone is truly loved and to disappointments on both sides of a relationship. It can also result in unmet expectations and lost opportunities for finding out who one's partner really is.

These are generalizations, of course. As human beings, we contain all of these potentials. It is very rare that someone will embody a pure yang or yin energy; we are combinations of both, and those parts of our nature respond to different stimuli, regardless of whether our brain is wired male or female. However, we generally don't have the opportunity to discover what our own balance is—our authentic sexual self—largely due to the fact that we are not allowed our innocence in which to do so.

We are all being set up, men and women alike, and I find this very sad. It is why my last holdout in terms of screening media for my teenage daughter (to the extent that I was able) was the graphic sexual content in Hollywood movies, even above edgy thematic material or violence. I wanted her to be able to have her own experience someday, untainted by those images and expectations. I had also hoped to teach her that her pleasure belongs to her, originates with her, and is not someone else's to give. If girls knew their own bodies and their own pathways to pleasure before becoming sexually active, they would not end up feeling that they are dependent on someone else to feel this way, and that they are somehow wanting because an insecure teenager, who is likewise ignorant, deals with their own insecurities by telling them so.

Studies show that the teenage brain is notoriously inaccurate at interpreting emotional cues. Almost 50 percent of the time, teens will misinterpret what emotion a facial expression is conveying. Add to that the inordinate pressure that teenagers are under today and it is a recipe for emotional meltdown in young relationships. However, the expectations that are laid down in these early relationships set the stage for later periods of our lives.

We tend to line things up according to our expectations. If our early experiences create expectations that we will not be attractive to the opposite sex, that we are not or will not be sexually competent, or that sex is shameful, and we have inept first experiences that don't stack up to our Hollywood expectations, it can have a lifelong impact on our future sexuality, even when as adults we "know better."

Leaving aside more extreme cases, where a girl might have been sexually or physically abused or exposed to sexual trauma of some sort, the range and colors of sexual expression that develop in a woman's life are so varied as to beg the question of what is "normal." Pretty much everything, if you ask me. If a woman is comfortable and consensual with her sexuality and sexual practices, then this is "normal."

The possibility for discovering an authentic sexuality was beautifully described to me by my client Grace. Grace had both the innocence and the opportunity to discover her own authentic sexuality. She spoke with gratitude of her first lover and how this happened for both of them. (And she later received thanks from one of this man's future girlfriends, for helping to create such a wonderful lover!)

Grace had been brought up in what she considered a somewhat sexually repressed family, so she said she carried the potential for ambivalence about sex and not fully opening to her sexuality. However, her first lover was also a virgin, enthusiastic, playful, and seemingly not filled with concern over his own ego needs to "look good." They began as innocents on an adventure together, not ready for intercourse in the beginning, so just exploring with each other what was possible. (Does this feel good to you? Do you like this? Wow, I didn't know *this* would happen. You think that's beautiful? Really?) They both felt it important to take time and go slow, to be ready before they took the next step, and there was a sense of safety between them.

Grace told me they made beautiful and very satisfying love for nine months before they decided to move to the next step and begin having sexual intercourse. By that time, she said it was "just one more dish at the feast." It wasn't the goal or the "destination" of their lovemaking, like she has experienced with other lovers since. Our ability to be in the moment and see which way the path will lead expands our experience and "range," and also allows us to authentically participate at any given time, without self-observation or distance.

Going Deeper

How Your Sexuality Emerged

One of the more important things we can do, if we want to come to an authentic sexuality, is to look at the cultural influences and early contexts that informed our sense of our sexual self. It may be hard to remember back before the messages started coming, because most came very early. Some of this material may have come up for you in your earlier exploration, but I suggest taking a deeper dive here, if you can.

- Was your caregiver comfortable with bodies? Bodily fluids?

- Were you made to feel ashamed of your body or that you were "dirty"?

- In what ways were you encouraged to explore what your body could do? Be active? Explore the limits of your body or environment? Or were you held back from this?

- Were you given negative messages about your body? What were they? From whom?

- Were there cultural, religious, or family myths you came up against that worked against you when you began to emerge as a sexual being? What were they?

- Was there any sexual trauma, experienced or observed, that impacted your first experiences? How did this affect you? Does it affect you still?

- What are your first memories of thinking of yourself as a sexual being—that your body would be in relationship to others sexually?

- Did you feel prepared for what was going to happen? How did that affect your early experiences?

- During your first sexual encounters, did you feel comfortable being seen? Being present in your body? Or were you self-observing?

- Did your partner seem interested in your experience, your pleasure, or just their own? How did they show you this?

- Did you talk to your partner about your experience and what felt good, or did you just expect them to know?

The issues brought forward in this chapter are similar to those in the last, but more specific to your sense of yourself as a sexual being and how you will be received as such. Early experiences with our sexuality live in us and inform our choices, even if we are not aware of them. Becoming aware will allow us more freedom to express ourselves authentically.

Once again, talk with your partner, if you have one, about your earliest experiences and ask them about theirs. If you have trouble bringing some of this material up, look at old pictures, watch old movies, read books that were important to you as your sexuality emerged. What did you see as romantic? What templates and expectations were laid down? See what the messages were in those movies and books and if they still live in you somewhere. See if this material is still up to date for you. What are you drawn to now?

It is also illuminating to talk with close women and men friends about *their* early experiences of being sexualized in our culture and whether they felt prepared for this. Notice whether there are similarities to yours. The more we discuss these things with others, the more it normalizes these experiences for all of us.

Chapter 11

The Body Electric— the Energetic Nature of Sex

No woman gets an orgasm from shining
the kitchen floor.   —Betty Friedan

While it might seem a bit of a side trip to go into the
nature of sexual response here, I have found that many
women, even at midlife, are still confused as to how
their bodies are made to work and why their sexual experiences are
not as satisfying as they would like them to be. In addition to looking at how our sexuality emerges, I think it is also worth exploring
what we can do to increase our satisfaction with this part of our
lives. We want to step into the next phase of our lives whole, and
our sexual selves are a huge part of that.

We are, at essence, electrical beings. The nervous system, which
sends signals to the brain and then back out to tell our foot to
move or our hand to close around an orange, is nothing but elec-
tricity carrying messages back and forth from point A to point B.
Everything we do is controlled by or enabled by electrical signals
running through our bodies.

It is no accident that when speaking of sexual attraction, we
talk of an electrical charge between people. There are those who

believe (and I am one of them) that sex is one way the human body can balance its electrical charge—recharge the battery, so to speak; get a tune-up—and the female is akin to a transformer in this scenario. The female receives energy from the male, transforms it, then gives it back. If both partners honor the other and the transaction, the process happens as the filling of a vessel, which then spills over in an abundance of ecstatic energy. This is a basic principle of Tantra, as it applies to sex—a way to bring two frequencies into alignment, at-one-ment, in the physical and subtle bodies, where sexuality is a doorway to the Divine. However, if our circuits are not open to receive, and we are outside self-observing, this cannot happen. The ability to be present is key.

Libido

Lack of libido is high on the list of almost every woman I see in my practice, especially at menopause. While stress is a huge component of this issue, it is important to ask, "What arouses us?" What opens our circuits and starts the flow of that life force that adds to our aliveness? Because almost to a one, these women are talking about being shut down, and not just sexually.

Is it a matter of needing novelty? Have we become so entrenched in the day-to-day rhythm of our lives that we are numb? Do our partners seem so overly familiar to us that we have lost interest in them as people? Have we lost interest in our own lives or disassociated from them? Are we physically exhausted? Are our hormones so out of balance that we can no longer run the machinery of desire, even when we are interested? Any or all of these are possibilities. It is equally possible that a woman may be entering a time in her life where it just feels more authentic to take a break, to be celibate for a while, which is an equally valid and growthful choice, but again, one for which she is made to feel "abnormal" in our overly sexualized culture.

What is libido really? Is it just sexual desire or more of an overall aliveness, a desire for life? The early twentieth-century psychotherapist Carl Jung used the word *libido* to include basic life force, and I tend to agree. All the machinery of desire might be online and functioning, but if the interest in life—the overall level of aliveness—is low, there will be no desire and no arousal.

Arousal, in a sexual sense, is the result of anything emotional, mental, or physical that a person finds erotic. During arousal, our heart rate, breathing rate, blood pressure, and alertness increase. The tone of certain muscle groups also increases. A man's penis will become erect and a woman's labia and vagina will swell and begin to produce lubrication.

What we find arousing or erotic is, of course, very subjective, and as we have seen, the template for it can be laid down very early in life. The variety in humans is endless in terms of what stimulates us, what we respond to, the conditions in which we find ourselves in our lives, and what we imprinted on in the past. All of these things influence our arousal. This is what is meant when we say that 90 percent of sexual arousal is between our ears.

We can all remember a time when we have anticipated being with a lover. Maybe we have been separated by a trip, or even just a day at the office. We begin to think about our lover, picture our meeting, visualize how our time will unfold. We may hear our beloved's voice on the phone. The arousal happens before we are even in each other's physical presence. Our body is fully alive, and we are practically orgasmic before we walk in the door. On the other hand, if there are a million things on our mind, our lover can be standing in front of us naked with a rose between their teeth and we hardly notice. It makes a difference.

For women in terms of arousal, it also very much makes a difference as to how we are approached. A common complaint of women is that men move too fast, that they are too direct in their approach and practice premature penetration. Men are often focused on the goal of intercourse, and they assume that a woman's libido and arousal are similar to their own (for which they can be forgiven if they received their sexual education from Hollywood). Remember, a woman will be more ready for and more open to sex if she feels safe, relaxed, and connected first. For a man, the connection often comes as a result of sex and the oxytocin surge that comes with it.

Each person has their unique balance of yin and yang erotic energy—the yang desiring directness, assertiveness, intense touch, or playfulness; the yin desiring receptiveness, passivity, gentle touch, and softness. As a rule, though, for a woman's body to become fully aroused during sexual contact, a lover should work their way from the outside in: using the voice and light touch; starting in less sensitive areas such as the face, neck, breasts, belly, and thighs; stroking in a way as to soothe and create safety, and only working toward sensitive parts as the woman's arousal becomes stronger. If you are looking for a full response, penetration with fingers, toys, or penis shouldn't happen until a woman has begun to naturally unfold and lubricate, to invite you in.

Remember, we are electrical beings. If our lover heads straight for the genitals and just tries to build a charge there, then the release will generally be smaller, more tightly focused, and *only* from there, where the charge is built. If the whole body is aroused first and the charge builds everywhere, then the release will be in the whole body as well. So, for the most full orgasm, allow for full arousal. To push that process and to be too focal or goal-oriented inhibits the building of the energy and mutes the release. Don't get me wrong—"quickies" can be highly erotic as well, but the charge is usually built before the sexual contact happens in that case. This is just a general truth in terms of the arousal of the female body.

Angels in the Architecture

Men often assume that women like to be touched in the same ways that they do, that what arouses them will also arouse their female partners. However, the difference in the sex organs alone argues against this. The penis is an external organ, covered with epidermis, the same kind of skin found elsewhere on the body. While sensitive, it can easily tolerate strong touch and friction, and many men enjoy and depend on this for arousal.

A woman's reproductive organs are internal. The outer lips of the vulva are covered with the same sort of skin as the penis, but the inner lips and the vagina, clitoris, and cervix are made up of mucus membrane, which is far more sensitive, needs to be kept wet (no thrusting of dry fingers inside!), and doesn't tolerate friction well until arousal is well underway. Mucus membrane is exquisitely sensitive, and if handled too soon or too roughly, can be very uncomfortable at worst and annoying at best, which will cause the woman's arousal cycle to shut down. For the best response, one should wait until moderate to full arousal has occurred before stimulating that tissue. Sensitive structures should be the last thing touched and certainly not penetrated until full arousal has been achieved. Readiness is everything.

Once we're fully aroused, we can hang out and play there or move on to orgasm. At this point, heart rate and circulation are increased and tissues are erect and swollen, in both men and women. Women have a very similar process to men in terms of the changes to their sexual organs during arousal. Many women are not aware of this, given that we teach the anatomy of our organs at best but not how to use them or how they function.

We are familiar with the erect penis; it has been an icon in art, architecture, and culture through the ages. However, women have erectile tissue as well, identical to men, and during arousal it also engorges and swells, protecting more delicate structures, such as the urethra, from injury during intercourse and decreasing the size of the vaginal opening to allow for more friction.

Moderate to full arousal, when the erectile tissue is engorged, is the time when more forceful touching and penetration can occur and not cause discomfort. In fact, many women desire this and need it to bring them to orgasm. However, it is important to communicate with your partner, because it can differ greatly between women as to when or even *if* they want more forceful touching or whether they can tolerate their clitoris being touched at all.

The clitoris gets lots of press, and we have all heard about how important it is. However, it is a very, very sensitive structure. The clitoris is protected by a covering of skin called the hood, in the same way that the glans of an uncircumcised penis is covered by the foreskin. These are analogous structures. They begin the same in all fetuses and then grow and develop differently depending on whether the fetus will become male or female. The clitoris is attached to the muscles of the inner labia, and while the sensation can be exquisite when the lips of the vulva are manipulated or tugged during penetration, sometimes directly touching the clitoris can be too much. Again, moving from outside to inside, palming and giving pressure but allowing the woman to decide how much and when she is open to more, will get the best results. If there is too much too quickly, the need to protect kicks in and a woman will shut down on some level.

When moderate to full arousal has taken place, and a woman's body is ready to receive penetration, lubrication will be enhanced, muscles in the pelvis will contract, and the cervix will literally lift up out of the way so that it will not be bumped with deep penetration (a significant cause of pain during sex for many women). Also at this point, the vestibular bulbs (a set of erectile tissues just underneath the outer labia that surround the opening of the vagina) plump up and engorge. These are connected as well to the shaft of the clitoris, so that every time they are rubbed or stimulated, they also stimulate the clitoris. Since everything is connected, there are many ways to stimulate the clitoris and create pleasure without ever touching the head of the clitoris itself. Many men are taught to go right for the clitoris, since it is the "hub of pleasure." However, this will generally be uncomfortable for a woman unless she is significantly aroused already. Full arousal is usually accomplished by subtler means. Essentially stimulating any of the structures around it will relay that stimulation to the clitoris.

When in touch with and open to one's partner and to enjoying the journey rather than being goal-oriented, moving too fast, and heading straight for the orgasm, it is possible to prolong this high arousal state for quite some time and, in so doing, extend your pleasure. Even if you have been having sex for decades, it is definitely worth adopting a "beginner's mind" and exploring what really feels good to you and your partner, with no goal in mind.

The Story of "Oh"

Orgasm, the muscle contractions that release and resolve the heightened state of arousal, is the destination for most lovers. It should be no surprise that during orgasm, we are flooded with our old friend oxytocin, the "love" hormone, and this helps us to feel bonded to our partner. In other words, orgasm is the result of and pleasurable release of all of this built-up energy and sexual arousal.

For most of us, orgasm is the goal of it all, and for some women, it seems like the Holy Grail because it's so elusive, given that they have not had the opportunity to come to full arousal first. For all that we are made to do it naturally and easily, many women are unable to achieve orgasm at all, or are not satisfied with the ones they have. For orgasm to occur, the process needs to unfold naturally, in safety and comfort. We need to be fully involved and not self-observing, and the charge needs to be built up sufficiently to have something to release. Much of the context in which women are having sex works against this.

Given the context in which we emerge as sexual beings in this culture, women often arrive at first sexual activity with a lack of self-knowledge as to what their path to orgasm is, a lack of sexual competence, and partners who know next to nothing about how the female body and brain actually work. Even though we are currently steeped in sex—it is used to sell literally everything—until recently our society was fairly sexually repressed. (Some would argue that it still is, underneath the racy veneer.) Most girls arrive at their first sexual experience believing that orgasm is their partner's gift to give, and if she doesn't have one, there is something wrong with her and she is not responsive, not that it might be her partner's lack of knowledge or skill.

Some couples luck out and, like my client Grace, their first experiences are safe and enjoyable, even adventurous, and they get better from there. However, my experience talking with women over the last few decades leads me to believe that most women end up settling for what they get and then feel that it is all they *can* get. Or maybe they are just the ones who talk about it, and all of those women for whom things are great don't feel the need to.

We don't think of the ability to orgasm as something we can learn, and we are generally not comfortable receiving assistance with something so private or that cuts so close to the bone of our self-esteem. However, the ability to orgasm or to have multiple orgasms is a learnable skill and there are some great teachers out there right now.

It is not the scope of this book to go into all of the details of the many ways and directions this learning can take place, but it is easy enough to explore and see what feels good to you, what arouses you (remember, arousal first, direction second), and what takes you in the direction of orgasm. Once you know this, you can practice, enjoy, and share your knowledge with your lover for the benefit of you both.

While Western medicine sees orgasm as a genital phenomenon, Nature is much more creative than that. We are wired for arousal and pleasure throughout our whole body, and whole-body orgasms are not only possible, especially for women, but known since ancient times. As far back as 400 BCE, humans were writing about sexuality and arousal.

The *Kama Sutra*, which most modern people think of as a manual containing sixty-four types of sexual acts and one hundred different sexual positions, is far more than that. It is a guide to virtuous and gracious living and the arrangement of a harmonious household and family life, including a section that reads like the Emily Post of the ancient world—proper protocol for engaging in social interactions and relationships. It addresses body, mind, and spirit. However, it also contains much practical advice on arousal techniques, role-playing, desire, and positions for sexual union.

This work lets us know that it was well known in the ancient world that we are wired throughout our body for ecstatic pleasure. In many, many cultures, sexual union is seen as a doorway to the Divine, which is much different than in our current Western culture, where sex is mostly seen as "getting off."

Women and men are also wired differently in terms of orgasm and *resolution*. Since a maintainable erection is necessary for a man to carry out the sex act and deliver his sperm, his arousal happens in such a way that blood flow is allowed into the penis, trapped there in order to maintain his erection, and then resolves with ejaculation. A resting period is necessary before he is able to achieve another erection. This resting period can last anywhere from fifteen minutes to twenty-four hours, depending on age and other factors.

Since the reproductive system of a woman is all interconnected, and her erectile tissue is able to engorge without trapping the blood, it is possible for her to have multiple orgasms with no refractory period. Now, in my opinion, the concept of multiple orgasms has also been used to browbeat women and make them feel that if they don't experience them, they are somehow wanting; and many things can be meant by this term, given the potential for full-body arousal and release. Becoming multi-orgasmic is something that can be learned if you want to, but you can have a very satisfactory sex life without it. Remember, the brain is a habit-forming organ. If you pair pleasure with certain stimuli often enough, you will lay down new pathways to pleasure, and whatever is good for you is . . . good and "normal."

Menopause is a great time to rediscover our bodies, since much is changed, and open up communication with our partners, whose bodies are likely also changing. If the sexual journey becomes one of mutual discovery, sex in the second half of life can be the best ever.

Going Deeper

Your Sexual Journey

I am certain that most women reading this have a good sense of what works and doesn't work for them sexually, even if they are not comfortable talking with their partners about it. As before, feel free to use this section in the way that feels most comfortable to you. Allow for time, so that you are not rushed and thoughts can float to the surface. Some of this you have already begun to explore. Again, if you feel that engaging with these questions may bring up material that is disturbing to you, explore with a therapist.

However you might choose to interact with this section, look with a bold eye and chart the path that brought you to the present time. By being fully present, you have a place from which to step off into your future.

Consider the following questions:

- What are some of the early images or messages about sexuality that you took in as being true?

- Was there a sense of ease about bodies in your home growing up or was that kept very private whether or not it was seen as shameful? How was this communicated?

- How old were you when you first saw someone of the opposite sex naked? Did it seem natural or was there a sense of shame or discomfort involved?

- What are your first memories of arousal? How did this primarily play out? Were they fantasies or feelings in your body or both?

- When did you have your first crush?

- What did your parents' level of affection with each other teach you? Were they comfortable being affectionate in your presence?

- Were you ever aware of them having sex or was that always when you were not around? How did it make you feel if you were aware of what they were doing?

- At what age did you first learn about sex? How? Was it a conversation with a parent, a class in school, a movie or media source, friends?

- As you got older, did you feel that you would be attractive to potential sexual partners? How did this sense develop? Was it through messages from family or friends, or comparing yourself to what you saw in the media?

- What were your first sexual experiences like? With whom? At what age? Did you feel forced or pressured?

- Were these early experiences safe and pleasurable or not? Were you made to feel shame? Fear? Both of these can shut you down, immediately and deeply.

- Did you ever have sex because you felt you "had" to, in order not to be considered a tease? Or in order to keep yourself safe? Or to fit in? In what way did this color your future experiences?

- Were you aware of your own pathway to pleasure before you began to engage with another or was that developed in conjunction with a partner? Is that something you have ever discovered?

- Have you explored your pathway to pleasure on your own, or only with a partner? Did you find anything different? Sometimes we think, *This is the way it is*, in terms of what we can experience in sex, because this is all we know. How much exploring have you done? Are you comfortable exploring?

- Do you generally allow enough time for arousal?

- Are you being touched in the way you want to be touched? If not, how would it be different if you were?

- What has been your most consistent frustration with sex? What might you do to change that?

- Was there a time when it was *exactly* the way you wanted it? What were the qualities of that experience?

- Do you feel that you embody an authentic sexuality or has it been largely framed by outside sources? If so, which sources?

Even if you think you are already aware of your pathway to arousal, take a little time to see what is present for you now and whether there might be more or something different at this point in your life. Share your findings with your partner. Ask them to share what arouses them. Once you have determined this, spend some time engaged in those activities, either alone or with your partner. Experiences of arousal don't need to be specifically sexual. Cooking a meal together, giving your partner a bath, or watching them do something they love may do this for you. If there is anything in your sexual life together that is uncomfortable for you, share that as well. Find each other in present time. The state of our libido, our *life force*, is key here. If we are shut down, very little may be arousing to us.

If you wish to explore more about authentic sexuality or work on this as a couple, or if you are interested in learning more about orgasm, consider looking online for teachers and classes that you can take in the privacy of your own home.

Chapter 12

Sex at Midlife

Sex doesn't disappear, it just
changes forms. —Erica Jong

A woman's experience of sex after menopause can be very
different from what it was in earlier years, for a variety
of reasons. Because of this difference, women often feel
that they are "not what they used to be" or that something is not
"right" or normal in their bodies. Many women are worried about
whether they will ever have "it" back. In fact, it is not uncommon
for postmenopausal libido and sexuality to be an enhanced experience. However, our cultural view of menopause is such that the
sense of loss is paramount, so changes are often seen as negative and
permanent. There are also women who are happy to "hang up their
spurs," so to speak, but feel pressure to continue to be interested in
sex because it is expected of them by their partners or peers.

As with sexuality in general, sexuality after menopause runs the
whole gamut in terms of diversity. The difference is not necessarily
one of lack, however. We can adjust to new ways of being sexually
just as we do in other areas of our lives as we grow and mature, and
the result can be a richer, more authentic sexuality than what we
had even when we were younger. Where you go with it is entirely
up to you and in your control.

Several factors inform this sense of difference that women feel.
Some are physical, such as lower levels of sex hormones and in

a different balance to each other, physical limitations that might restrict sex positions, or changes to the vaginal tissue due to loss of estrogen that make it less elastic and sex less comfortable than it once was. Arousal time is also delayed after menopause. (It generally takes about twenty minutes longer for a postmenopausal woman to reach full arousal than a premenopausal one.)

Other factors are more psychological or emotional, such as being in long-term relationships with little that seems new or stimulating anymore or a belief that one is no longer attractive as one ages. For a woman who has spent a couple of decades raising children (and sometimes a husband), everything changes when the nest is empty. She feels like she has stepped into a whole new life and the landscape is quite different.

My client Karen felt very liberated by this. She and her husband embarked on a second honeymoon that lasted for years. It didn't just happen; they decided to be young and sexy again and do the things they used to enjoy. It is just as likely, and just as normal, for a woman to decide at this juncture that she wants to have a period of celibacy in order to take stock of her life, land where she is, and put her energy into the newly stimulated creative centers of her brain, in order to birth the next phase of her life.

With the reproductive urge no longer driving the brain and a new perspective of life opening up, many women choose to engage in sexual relationships of a different kind. They take up more casually with a sexual partner rather than being in a "relationship," or perhaps they become sexual with women for the first time. It might make sense to them, during this time of integration and honoring authenticity, to be with someone wired more similarly to themselves.

Studies suggest that sexual response can be quite different for women who are in long-term relationships than for those in early stages of intimacy, and many postmenopausal women find themselves in this position, with decades-old marriages or partnerships.

According to the studies, the sexual response of women in long-term relationships more commonly stems from a need for intimacy rather than a need for sex, as it often does for men or for women in the hormone-driven phase of new relationships. In long-term relationships, especially when the distractions and fatigue associated with children are present, a woman often moves toward sex for other reasons, such as a partner's need, a need for closeness or the help of a partner, or some other reward that is important to her, rather than a desire for sex. Or a woman might experience arousal when she engages in fantasy, reads a romantic book, or watches a movie, but not at the end of a long day when her partner is interested in sex. Her need may be for arousal but not the sex itself.

It becomes critically important at this juncture to be able to communicate with our partners, to engage in a dialogue that lets them know where we currently find ourselves in this process and that our loss of interest is not personal, if that is the case. If a relationship is to last through many years, it will pass through multiple phases—and these *are* phases. If we are truly alive and present, change is the only constant.

As mentioned before, I think of libido more in the Jungian sense of life force—which includes sexual libido—rather than as a term for sexual desire, as it has come to be more commonly used. The two are very much intertwined, however, and the women I work with suffer from lack of both; one derives from the other. This is not surprising, given the level of stress we live under in our current culture.

Finding Each Other Again

In most modern relationships, we have come to live on parallel tracks to our partners; we have different schedules, different deadlines, and different responsibilities. This creates a lack of intimacy—truly, a lack of a shared life. Communication distills down to housekeeping details and dealing with the children or pets, or trying to coordinate the schedules of both partners. Often the only time that we are in close enough physical proximity to our lover for sex to be possible is at the end of a very long day, when we fall into bed exhausted.

Now, for men, this is usually not a problem. Remember, men are wired visually. They can generally be ready to go pretty quickly, and they derive relaxation and release from having sex. For women, it is the opposite. Women need intimacy and connection in order to open, to want to have sex. If the laundry list of the undone is running through a woman's head, or even if she is merely exhausted, the last thing she generally wants is to have to deal with what feels like someone else's needs. Sex feels like one more thing on the to-do list. (Though sex should nourish both parties, a woman is more likely to view sex as a chore when she is distracted or exhausted.)

Often the way that we engage in sex also takes on a similar parallel quality to the rest of the shared life. With the intimacy being lost, sex becomes routine and each partner is likely to fall into an internal rather than a shared experience. We go to sex looking for intimacy, but in actuality, intimacy needs to be the ground of being for sex if it is going to be a shared experience.

If we are going to have a vibrant sexuality into our later years, it is important that we make sure it is authentic to who we are today, where we are now. It is important to tease out what is truly pleasurable for us, what *we* desire, as opposed to what is expected of us because of our age or by our family or culture. So many women have never explored their own desire because their ideas about this were shaped at an early age by parental or religious expectations, an immature partner, Hollywood, or porn. For example, we might be ashamed if what we desire deviates from the cultural norm and involves kink or fetishism. Many women choose to explore this at midlife.

It is also true that what we desire, need, or want now may be very different from what it was when we were younger, even if we were authentic in our sexuality in younger years. Finding ourselves at a different stage of our lives—with different goals, roles, and hormone balance—it is a perfect time to check in and update where we find ourselves sexually.

Very often a client will come into my office with the concern that her male partner wants sex much more than she does, and there must be something wrong with her. She still loves him but just has no interest. She continues to "do it" but not as often, and she finds no pleasure in the act. She does this because she fears he will leave her if she doesn't.

Having sex when you don't want to, when it is uncomfortable, or "just to keep things stable" doesn't feel good for either partner and often ends up separating a couple more. Sex is an energy exchange and when one person is not present, it is always evident. It is so important to stay in the present moment. If we are in any way living in the past, watching ourselves from a distance, afraid of judgment, or even just doing it the same way all of the time, we will lose our energy for it.

I am always surprised when I ask such a client if she has spoken to her partner about this and she says no. There is a lot of shame wrapped up in this for women. They feel if they are not perpetually "ready" for sex, then they fail as women and no one will want them. This is yet another of the insidious legacies of the type of sex portrayed by Hollywood and in porn. It is important to open up and communicate with our partners what is going on with us. When we do, we'll often find that many of them are going through something similar.

Going Deeper

Your Authentic Sexual Self

Knowing where we came from as sexual beings and what experiences helped to shape us and frame our viewpoint is important. Many women find that all of these things change as they hit midlife: how they frame their sexuality, what they want from it, how it feels physically, why they want what they want. This section will ask you to stand aside a bit from where you *have* been and look with a clear eye at where you are *now*, what is important *now*, what is authentic for you *now*. You may not readily know. If that is the case, here's an opportunity to begin to explore.

Try to give each question a little time. See what has changed. Are you okay with the changes? Or do you feel that what you were is better somehow, and this is a loss? Sexual energy is life force, so if yours is diminished, in whatever way you channel it, your vibrancy will diminish as well. Tell yourself the truth.

- When you were younger, did you ever question or creatively explore what you *really* wanted in regard to sex or did you accept that what you experienced was what there was?

- What is the state of your libido at this time of life? How does this compare to when you were younger?

- What sexual activities would you like to experience or fantasies would you like to explore but do not indulge in? Why not? What is one step you could take to bring you closer to where you want to be?

- What do you deny in your sexuality? What do you want that you "shouldn't" want?

- If you are with a partner, how does your libido compare with theirs? Does one of you want sex or engage with life more than the other? Do you talk about it in a way that feels nourishing to you both or is there a lot of blaming?

- Why do you have sex at this time in your life? For pleasure? Security? To feel needed or connected? To be in control? To feel "normal"? How successful is sex in actually delivering this to you?

- How do you want the experience of sex to make you feel? What do you go to sex for?

- Where is sex on your list of *what you really want* right now? Are there other creative outlets that you prefer to give your energy to?

- Is the power dynamic relatively equal in your relationship? Is it different around sex than other areas of the relationship?

- Do you feel like you can speak honestly with your partner about your needs and what you want? If not, why not?

Many marriages and relationships fail at midlife. Often children are leaving the home at the same time a woman is being re-created through the metamorphosis of menopause. The hormonal trance that has kept her in service to reproduction and putting everyone else ahead of herself on her to-do list has passed. She is now being impulsed toward her creativity and authenticity. Couples that thrive into their elder years are open to reevaluating, adjusting, and planning *together* for a joint future.

This chapter has asked you to look at how your sexual needs and desires have changed at midlife. Hopefully knowing about the underlying hormonal and stress-related changes that impact this has helped you to normalize this. In this chapter, you have been asked to reevaluate the sexual aspect of your life, or your lives together as a couple, and to explore how to embody your authentic sexuality going forward. Create space for this, either alone or as a couple, if you are partnered, and get to know each other again, *where you are now*. What is true for each of you?

It is easy to hold an image of someone frozen in the past, particularly if you are living parallel lives now. Discuss your needs, wants, and desires. Discuss how things might have changed and what you want to create *together* going forward that honors this. If you feel you need outside help, it is a great time to find a couples counselor. This helps many couples, even if everything seems to be working well in their relationship, as it creates a space for just listening and working with these issues.

Chapter 13

Creating Good Sex

Seduce yourself first. —Kamand Kojouri

M any women, when they are honest with themselves for the first time, find that they are a long way from where they truly want to be in regard to sex. They are either meeting someone else's timetable or needs or, having been raised when the subject of sex was somewhat taboo, they find they don't really know *what* they want. If you are at a loss, don't worry. You are not alone. If this is something that is important to you, it is just another journey of discovery. Even if you are clear about what you want, if you don't find yourself there, it is time to take the first step on the path to that destination. Here are some things to get you started. I am sure you will think of more once you get going.

Find Your Pathway to Pleasure

Sex, like any other relationship, begins with oneself. What do you want? You can't ask for it if you don't know. Are you worthy? Have you been shamed? Does a partner keep control over you by judging you and putting you down? What feels good to you? How do you get there? How do you want to express yourself? We have to give ourselves permission to be whole in order to be who we *truly* are. Giving ourselves permission to express our most authentic self gives others the opportunity to receive it and enjoy it. So, give yourself some time to see what feels good, what fantasies you like, what you want to wear, how you want to be received. Libido is life force. What makes you feel alive? The internal and external are deeply intertwined.

Also, look at what you believe to be true about this time of life. I believe the Mind to be a creative field. If we hold certain beliefs that are limiting, then we tend to line things up that way. We make choices that reflect that. Do the self-inquiry to catch up to present time. What do you feel about this time of life? Have you been made to feel that a woman's sexuality should "turn off" or end at a certain age? If so, you are more likely to find yourself winding down.

One of my clients, Elizabeth, came in with the concern that her husband wanted sex all the time and she no longer did. She decided to take the challenge to figure out what she really wanted at this time of life. She decided she did want to have sex but wanted it to make her feel more alive, not be a chore. She began by balancing her hormones, which gave her body the raw materials it needed. Then she embarked on discovering what gave her sexual pleasure. She took time by herself, without her husband, to figure this out. During this time, she was not sexual with him. She then took the risk to talk with him honestly about what she had found out and to ask for what she needed. He was thrilled, because he knew that sex wasn't great for her and he had felt the burden of trying to figure out what would make her happy.

This is huge, because most of us, if we are honest with ourselves, think that if our partner is "the one," they will magically know what we need and bring it out of us. We bring significant baggage to bed with us that limits our expression and enjoyment, but our partners rarely know what is going on. If we take the risk to show ourselves, it frees our partner to enjoy it and to do the same.

For Elizabeth, sex became enjoyable again—because it was authentic and truly met her needs—and then she couldn't get enough! Her husband had a hard time keeping up with her after that and that became the complaint (which really wasn't a complaint).

Take a Fresh Look at Your Partner

Your partner is likely going through many of the same emotional and physical changes that you are. We tend to think of people as snapshots in time and relate to them that way, rather than seeing the ways in which they change from day to day. Particularly if our attention is focused in a different place than our partner on a daily basis, this is easy to do, and why so many people form intimate relationships with people in their workplace—they have shared interests and occupy the same space at the same time. They know and see the "current version" of that person.

In modern life, we are often living on parallel tracks to our partners, with different jobs, focuses, schedules, responsibilities. We tend to communicate around household issues or children and lose touch with what it is that is currently making our partner vibrant and alive.

Create some time and space to catch up to present time with your partner, see what fills their days and emotional space, what they are thinking about. Share what is going on with you. Talk about what you would like to move toward in your life *together*. Set some mutual goals that you can work toward together. If there is anything I have seen over and over again in life, it is that all of our secrets are really the same secret. Once we start sharing what is happening for us, there is generally mutual ground to inhabit. Men go through a midlife andropause and are often experiencing similar things, but they also have a cultural expectation to be different.

Address Any Physical Issues

Many postmenopausal women, or their partners, are on medications that can affect sexual desire or sexual function (the ability to create and maintain an erection or to have an orgasm). Examples of these include antidepressants, antianxiety medications, blood pressure medications, cholesterol-lowering medications, diuretics, and medications for acid reflux and ulcers. If you are on any of these medications and experience difficulty with desire or response, check with your health-care provider to see if there are lifestyle changes you can make to reduce your need for the medication or if there are other medications you can use that carry fewer of these kinds of side effects.

A general improvement in your health and reducing the number of medications you are taking will have a positive effect on sexual desire and response. Reduce any pain you might be in and work to reverse symptoms of diabetes and heart disease. Physically, sexual response has a lot to do with our vascular system and how well blood is flowing. Many of the issues related to poor sexual response can be addressed through diet and moderate exercise. This is something you and your partner can work on together. Depression, lethargy, and obesity will also diminish sexual desire.

Check your hormone balance. Low levels of estrogen, progesterone, or testosterone can affect your desire to engage in sexual activity and your ability to have an orgasm. Low levels of estrogen can leave the vagina without elasticity, making for painful intercourse. This is very easy to fix; there is no reason any woman should suffer from painful intercourse due to vaginal "dryness" (which is really lack of elasticity, not dryness). Even most doctors of women with estrogen-positive cancers will allow treatment of the vaginal tissue, because it carries so little risk. The same is true for low adrenals and neurotransmitters. High or low levels of certain neurotransmitters can interfere with sexual function.

Finally, have fun and get creative with where you have sex, the time of day, or sexual positions. Do something new together! If you have physical limitations, such as painful knees, that keep you from enjoying some of the positions you enjoyed in your younger years, make friends with a chair! Using a chair or the edge of a bed can take the pressure off of painful knees. Making love in the water, whose buoyancy helps with issues of gravity, can bring new life back into a sexual relationship in more ways than one. Lie side by side, back to front. Get creative.

The novelty of new things—breaking out of old patterns—as well as the ways in which they can assist with issues of physical limitation can help to get the juices flowing again. As much as possible, bring your fantasies into real life.

Create Space for Intimacy

Make a date night. This is not necessarily for sex (though that may become a welcome side effect) but to get to know your partner again. What are they thinking about, focusing on? What makes *them* feel alive these days? Sharing our journeys creates intimacy. Men often experience changes in their libido and sexual capacity as a result of midlife hormone changes as well and are just as reluctant to talk about it due to the way they are acculturated. If you set the stage and open up the subject, you might be very surprised at what comes up. Speak frankly about where you find yourself in relationship to your own desire, pleasure, and goals. You may find that you and your partner are in a more similar place than you think. Then you can act on "making more" together.

Just having a time set aside each week to look forward to, just for enjoying yourselves, can create anticipation and eventually arousal, if you want to use your time that way. Creating intimacy in other ways will also enhance the sexual intimacy with your partner.

Create a container for communing with your partner by doing the things you used to enjoy together when you were courting or by sharing and enjoying new interests that have evolved. Get away from home and the pressure of all your responsibilities occasionally, if that is an option for you. Read a juicy book together; watch a movie you find erotic. Find your own personal joy (and the Beloved in yourself) and that will spill over into your relationship.

Be Aware of Your Expectations

It is very difficult to feel turned on by someone who just feels like another item on your to-do list, or by someone you are bored with (even if that is yourself), or with whom you are frustrated or angry most of the time because communication has disappeared. Remember, men and women often have unrealistic expectations of each other and of what it is reasonable to expect our partners to provide. Especially as women, we tend to expect our partner to be all things to us. For example, the male brain is wired in a more pragmatic, focused, "left brain" way, so a man might feel that he is being asked to fix a problem when all his partner wants to do is talk about her experience (her brain being wired more to find the connections in things). This can begin to feel overwhelming for men, feeling responsible to figure out how to "make it better" for their partner, and they will often shut down and back off of communicating rather than experience more of it.

Quite often women are expecting their men to provide types of emotional support and engagement and interest in romantic details that are better provided by a glass of wine and a good schmooze with a girlfriend. Both parties end up feeling frustrated, dissatisfied, and unappreciated or unloved when this is not the case.

Take time to identify what your expectations of your partner are, and ask yourself if they are realistic, especially in light of decreased time for intimacy. Also, be clear with your partner about these expectations. We often feel "they should know by now," but most people are not very good mind readers. Remember, too, that just because we have said we want or need something doesn't mean our partner is bound in some way to give it to us. We need to accept this.

Even more important is to approach our partner with interest and trust—curiosity—rather than expectation and dissatisfaction. If we are always coming only from our own perspective or talking about what is wrong, we are less likely to hear what the experience of our partner really is. We will just hear their anger or receive resistance to our perspective.

Many couples find it helpful to begin couples counseling at this stage of life, even if they feel nothing is really "wrong" with their relationship. In an environment set aside for the creation of communication and intimacy, you can acquire tools that will be carried forward into the second half of life to enrich the relationship.

Allow Time for Full Arousal

Remember falling in love: the hours spent looking into the eyes of our Beloved, holding hands, stroking their skin, talking (the voice of our Beloved is one of the most arousing things there is), making the connection? It helps to move back in this direction if we want to have a full sexual response, especially after menopause. (Remember, it takes a little longer.) Allowing for time to just be in each other's presence and build slowly is core to this process.

Make sure your partner knows this. Go for the full connection! Connection is all-important to the female brain and body. Turn off the cell phone and the computer. Make sure there will be no interruptions by children or pets. Create your own inviolable time and space. Our current technology has so habituated us to being available twenty-four hours a day that we don't even believe we deserve time to ourselves anymore.

Don't try to rush sex in the postmenopausal years. It is generally not the time for quickies or the "five-minute shag" just before you drop off to sleep—not if you want your partner to come back for more. However, couples do find that changing it up a bit—making time for sex in the morning, for instance, when both partners have more energy—can be very effective. A change of place can add excitement as well—anything that will break a stale pattern.

A Word about Pleasure: More

Most women who are currently in their menopausal years were not raised to focus on their own pleasure. Many may not even admit to having preferences or admit that their pleasure should be a priority. In fact, pleasure was a little bit of a dirty word when we were young. In my home, I heard a lot about responsibility, expectations, and appearances. I was not encouraged to have preferences, and when I did, I was taught to put them after the desires of others, to not be "selfish." When my mother asked me in college what my goals were, and one of them was to be happy, she was horrified. I know I am not alone in this.

Often women cannot even say what would bring them pleasure, much less do they engage in it; they just don't "go there." We make many excuses; by the time the rest of the to-do list is taken care of, we don't feel we have the leisure, the money, or the energy to engage in it. As science discovers more about how pleasure affects the body—boosting the immune system, flooding the brain with feel-good neurotransmitters that affect every system of our body—we begin to see how important it is that we take the time to learn about and practice pleasure. And I am not just speaking about sexual pleasure. Mother Nature wants us to be happy while we are here! It is part of the Plan. It is part of how our bodies stay healthy and our whole being thrives.

Not to mention that when we are awash in pleasure, it is contagious. Those around us benefit as well, and there is nothing more attractive than a woman at home with and enjoying herself! When a woman knows what makes her happy and is engaging in it, she sweeps others up into the same happy vortex. It is part of our tantric role as transformers. Our being happy takes a lot of pressure off of our partners, who are trying to figure out what to do to make us happy, so they are happier, too, and want to give us what we want!

Again, the media, which sells us culture, bears some responsibility for our lack of awareness as to what will really bring us pleasure. In our consumer-driven society, we are told that acquiring things will bring us pleasure. But is it true? According to the ads, if we just have the right car, have the right clothes, drink the right beer, or use the right toothpaste, we will be happy. I am old enough to remember when advertising campaigns first began to hit their stride. Their success literally depended on telling us how to feel, what to want, to see ourselves in a certain way. This sets up an endless seeking for the next "thing" that will make us happy—and it rarely does. Or if it does, it is very transitory.

In difficult economic times, pleasure takes a back seat to necessity if we buy the model that pleasure is the acquisition of things. However, no matter who we are or what our current economic status is, we can create pleasure at any time, in any place. It just requires being present. We will not be aware of the pleasure of sun on our skin, or the color red that blazes forth from a spring tulip, or the way our skirt swishes against our legs as we walk, if we are focused on our problems, or a fight with our spouse, or the fact that we are late to pick up the kids from school.

Again, there are many good teachers out there right now who are focusing on teaching how to access and experience pleasure; however, we often do not think to go out and learn about such intimate things from a teacher. We take what we have and just make that enough, make it okay, even if it is not. Today, with good online workshops on Tantra, sexuality, and pleasure available, and the fact that one can take basic courses on sexual anatomy and response in the privacy of one's own home, many men and women are moving forward as partners and learning together.

If You Need to Take a Break, Do . . .

In midlife, when our time of being strongly polarized as male or female for the purposes of reproduction is over, both men and women move back closer to hormonal center and begin the process of integration. As men and women, we each contain the masculine and feminine principles; one just tends to express more strongly than the other. Our life task in midlife is to find our authenticity, integrate the various phases and experiences of our lives, and become Wise Women, or elders.

Unlike my client Karen, who embarked on a second honeymoon, the urge toward sex diminishes for many women at midlife and other things begin to arise. When the sexual urge is no longer driving the train, the brain space and emotional space that was once used engaging in, analyzing, and agonizing over our sex lives opens up to make way for creativity, integration, and life-purpose activities. Our society doesn't support this—we are made to feel abnormal if we are not hot to trot all of the time, but in the natural process of maturation, it is very common for sex to take a back seat for a while. For many women, this means a period of celibacy.

We often think of celibates in religious terms—of those who are cloistered and have taken a vow, or those engaging in tantric celibacy practices. However, many women and men make the conscious choice to not have sex for a while, whether they are partnered or not. While this is more common at midlife, when the sexual urge is diminishing, many younger women and men are also taking a "time out" from sexual activity *because* the sexual urge is so strong and has taken over their lives. They feel carried away by the culturally supported need to "hook up" all of the time, and no longer find anything meaningful in it. As the interest in casual sex wanes, the choice for celibacy goes up. We are no longer interested in having sex with the wrong partner or just because it is expected of us.

There are many reasons we might make a conscious choice to be celibate for a period of time, and in making it a conscious choice, it can be very empowering. The erotic parts of ourselves inhabit the realm of the great Mystery, and are a journey to be explored. We don't often get the opportunity to do that in our current culture.

In taking a conscious break, we are gifting ourselves time and space to explore our feelings without necessarily having to act on them in conventional ways. This can free up time and energy to focus on goals or projects we are interested in—such as painting, writing, or taking stock of our lives. It could be to explore, if we are single, who we are authentically and who we might be authentically attracted to, without the confusion that sometimes comes from being swept up in sexual desire, only to find, once it begins to fade, that we are once again with the wrong person. As women, what we really want from sex is connection, and there is often sadness after the casual sex that is supported in our culture because that connection is lacking.

If we are in a relationship, it becomes very important to communicate our thinking and reasons for this choice to our partner so that it is understood and not seen as personal. They may even want to join us on this journey of self-exploration or focused attention. Don't be surprised, however, if a similar dynamic to the one that comes up in your conversations about sex (who wants more, who is more in tune, more spiritual, who is withholding) is eerily mimicked in your conversations about celibacy.

Once the charge around sex is removed, you might find a clearer path to explore in your relationship. This choice could be for a few weeks or months without sex, or even open-ended. It is not uncommon to find that, in the end, it actually recharges your libido.

So, once again, there is clearly a wide range of normal and a wide variety of reasons women might wish to seek or avoid certain sexual experiences after menopause. Catching up to ourselves in present time, learning what our authentic needs and desires are around sex becomes key—then we can communicate those to our partner so that we create more interest, trust, and curiosity, and we don't fall prey to unnecessary misunderstandings and hurt.

Whatever your past history and experience might be, pleasurable sexual experience can be in your future if you want it, and there is no better time to start than now. Full-body arousal and orgasm can be learned if you are willing to explore and open to new terrain. As mentioned, there are several wonderful teachers out there to guide you on this journey, but your best teacher is your own body! All the better if you have a willing and adventurous partner. Go forth! Enjoy!

Going Deeper

Taking Stock of Your Sexual Life

Midlife is a wonderful time to take stock. In earlier sections, you have explored what formed your sense of sexual self in the first place. In this section, I would like you to take a look at how this might have changed in midlife. Most of us think about ourselves in terms of our past. The task of this time of life is to take the time to catch up to the now, assess desires, and chart a path toward the future. If you can interest your partner in doing so as well, even better.

- What was the dynamic in your parents' marriage?
  Were they communicative partners? Did they seem to enjoy touch and physical intimacy?

- Where did your ideas of what a marriage or partnership *should* look like come from?

- In what ways might you be unconsciously carrying on a legacy from your family of origin, their expectations, or the expectations of the culture at large?

- What went into your choice of a partner in your earlier years? Good provider, good looks, someone "safe"? How might those needs have changed at this stage of life? What do you want now?

- If you are in a relationship or partnership, what needs are being met, and how? What needs are not being met? What are you getting out of the relationship, and why? How might you change this?

- Who are you dependent on? Who is dependent on you?

- In your relationship, who is in control of when, where, and how you have sex? Be honest.

- How do you and your partner share the dynamic of receiving or asserting control, dominance? If you don't, why do you think that is? True preference? Habit? One person's need to play a certain role?

- Do you engage in sexual activity more or less than you would actually desire? Why?

- Is sex satisfying for you now? Why or why not?

- Do you *know* what you really desire? Think about it. Write it down. What limits you from having what you desire?

- What, if anything, stops you from sharing this with your partner? Do they listen?

- Do you know what your partner desires, and are they able to express this to you?

- Have you ever contemplated "taking a break" from sex and being celibate for a while? If you did, were you partnered at the time? What did that time yield for you? Did your relationship survive? Get better or worse?

This chapter has given you some specific suggestions on how to address areas in your sexual relationship with your partner that might help you get back on the same page and look at what could work for you *now*. It may not be readily apparent to you what the problems are. Allow yourself time to really follow your feelings and intuitions about this.

If any of these suggestions call to you, try them out. Break the usual pattern. Take the steps you need to take to bring yourself into a place with your partner where the sexual exchanges between you feel true to you both. After identifying what you think can make things better, talk with your partner about what *they* feel needs to be addressed right now. Again, if you feel you would benefit from some outside help in this effort, set up some time with a couples counselor or go on a retreat for couples that addresses sexual communication.

PART THREE

Midlife Course Corrections

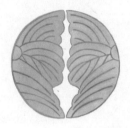

Chapter 14

Finding Our Way Home

Life should not be a journey to the grave with the intention of arriving safely in a pretty and well-preserved body, but rather to skid in broadside, thoroughly used up, totally worn out, and loudly proclaiming, "Wow, what a ride!" —**Hunter S. Thompson**

When I think about my life's journey, the image often arises of being in a small ship on the open sea, looking up at a field of stars and using them to show me the way home. The ancients navigated by signs from earth and sky, orienting themselves by the landmarks and stars that were their daily companions, in order to cross the unknown and reach their destination. When exploring uncharted seas, navigators would use instruments of celestial navigation to check their bearings several times a day to ensure that their ship remained on course.

Navigating a life is not unlike traversing an uncharted sea. Even today, we use companions and familiar landmarks to chart our journey. Following our life trajectory needs to be a fluid process because things can change moment to moment. Checking our bearings is a fluid process as well, and it is sometimes quite an unconscious one. However, when we find ourselves in uncharted waters, it is common to move toward the familiar, and this keeps us retracing old patterns, even if they may no longer be the most authentic to who we are now.

Checking our bearings and adjusting our course is not something we can do two or three times in a lifetime, at major milestones, and expect good results. Those who check in more frequently will benefit from being able to make the minor adjustments necessary to stay on course and remain authentic to the present, rather than having to make major adjustments later. It is easy to be knocked off course and to not even notice it, particularly since we are often swimming against a cultural tide that seems bent on distracting us, telling us how to feel and live our lives. We need to know who we are and what we want in order to keep our course true.

Midlife—menopause—is a perfect time to take our bearings and make any adjustments needed, for several reasons. First, our body supports us completely in this process. Our hormonal balance is changing, and our brain is being directly stimulated toward a different life task, moving us from a focus on reproduction, childrearing, and nurturing to that of our own creative endeavors. Second, for women who have children, the transition to an empty nest (which is a huge shift) usually dovetails closely with this change in hormonal status. Even if we don't have children, for most of us, our lives are changing in major ways, hormonally and relationally—everything is thrown up in the air—and it is a perfect time to decide how we want the pattern to re-form when everything lands again. We *do* have the power to determine that pattern and chart our own course.

We are in the chrysalis, becoming elders—the Wise Women of our world—and as such, we want to distill the wisdom we have gained to this point in our lives and begin to see how we are drawn to gift this wisdom and express our creativity going forward. If we don't know where we are heading, this time of change and transformation can feel deeply disruptive.

We must find our own North Star to navigate by, our own True North to which we can return time and again to get our bearings. That True North is our essential self. During the course of our lives, different "selves" have been authentic to the various phases we have lived through, and they made perfect sense for that period in time. We have inhabited different roles and seen ourselves through different lenses. It is important at this time to look back through these phases of our lives and identify the parts that make up our core self, that which we know to be essential to who we are and that we wish to bring forward with us into the next phase of life.

These qualities might reach all the way back to those of our early childhood—an innate joy and life force we expressed at three, our clear vision of what we loved at ten, the growing awareness of self and what our role was to be, that became clear in the teenage years. All of these are important parts of who we are, and they will continue to inform our journey. There are other roles and ways of seeing ourselves that are no longer relevant to the next phase of our lives, and these we can acknowledge, celebrate, or mourn and then allow to live in the past. They do not need to be brought forward in our journey.

The following chapters contain some explorations that will help you to find your True North, your essential self, so that you can chart the course of the second half of your life in a direction, and to a destination, that feels true to who you are now, not a previous version of yourself. The woman who owns and fully inhabits herself, without apology, is a force for grounding and change in the world. The truest version of ourselves is the destination. This is home.

The Mirror of Mortality

Midlife is a time during which we begin to face the reality that we are aging and will eventually die. This is difficult for many women—they find it hard not to stay stuck in the past, where things might not be what they truly want now, but are familiar. The first step to reorienting and making sure we are on course to our True North is to become disengaged from our *attachment* to the past and how things used to be. This includes accepting the physical changes. We begin to notice the signs of aging in our body more and more, and friends around us begin to pass on. I remember my grandmother saying to me when she was in her eighties that when she looked in the mirror, she was shocked at the stranger she saw there; that inside, she still felt like a sixteen-year-old girl. I was in my twenties at the time, so while I thought it poetic, I couldn't really understand what she was saying. At sixty, I did.

In my early forties, I often did not recognize the signs of aging in myself for what they were; I thought that something was just "off." How odd that the texture of my skin was changing or that my hair wasn't as thick as it used to be. What was I doing differently? Was I missing a nutrient? Was something wrong with me? What had changed? I canvassed the medical literature to find out what might be causing such changes. It was a while before it dawned on me that this was just the natural progression of things, that my body wouldn't be staying the way it "had always been." I was aging. Like most youthful creatures who deem themselves immortal, I had never really given much thought to how the process would begin to unfold or what the slow progress of aging might look like.

For many women, an initial reaction to these changes is to feel betrayed by their bodies, shortchanged, or as if they had been dealt a blow. It becomes paralyzing and takes up all of their psychic space and energy. Others can just joke about it and move on. However, with the gift of turning outward from our constant self-referencing (which follows naturally in the wake of brain and hormonal changes), we generally come to see that it is just the natural course of things, and we begin to adjust to the "new normal."

In the beginning, most of us will go back to old strategies that were successful in earlier stages of life, to try to address new physical challenges. However, many of the old strategies no longer work as we age, due to changes in the body's metabolic processes and hormonal balance. Some women become stuck in old strategies to the point of becoming obsessive and ineffective, often making the problem worse (as in the case of women with fatigued adrenals who eat significantly less and exercise obsessively, thinking it will help them lose weight).

Cherishing the Past

One of the most prevalent themes that emerges in my work with women during the menopausal years is the difficulty in leaving the past behind and being fully present in one's life during this transition. There are many reasons a woman might remain stuck in the past and be unable to come to present time while stepping through this doorway into the next phase of her life. To begin with, the past represents our lived experience and our competence. It is all we know. Sometimes it is the physical symptoms of menopause and the emotional changes that accompany them that drive women away from the present moment. They feel depressed, fatigued, and overextended, which makes all of the other symptoms worse, and it becomes difficult to feel positive about anything that is happening in their bodies and in their lives. It sometimes takes a little work with hormone balancing to begin to support the body enough that one can rise up out of the pit long enough to even see the road ahead and know what the lay of the land is.

Sometimes it is fear that sends us running for the past, to a previous identity that is well established and familiar. The known seems to us to be much safer than discovering what is authentic for us in the here and now. However, while it may seem safer, it also keeps us focused in the past and, consequently, to a certain extent, in fantasy.

It therefore uses up more energy and brings less satisfaction. It is not uncommon for women who find themselves oriented toward previous identities, and who have daughters who reach young womanhood during the women's midlife transition, to begin to live vicariously through their daughters. Some even find themselves in competition with them, consciously or unconsciously.

Most often, what drags us back is what I call "the weight of the undone," the things that we never allowed ourselves to fully experience or to mourn or celebrate. Germaine Greer, one of the major feminist voices of the mid-twentieth century, once said, "When we reach menopause, all that we dreamed and did not do often comes to reproach us, for having given ourselves away to others' expectations and needs. We often spend years doing this and then feel that, the sacrifice done, it is not even appreciated."

In order to live in the present, it is imperative that we cherish the past. We need to mourn what we never had or things that we never did. We need to celebrate the gifts life *did* bring our way. It is important to identify the things that have become essential to who we are—that are still authentic to us—and carry them forward into the next phase of life. The things that are no longer authentic to who we are now must be honored and left behind if we are to make this transition to living in present time.

How do we even begin to do this? As the old adage goes, "Getting old is not for the faint of heart." We must begin to engage in the process of sifting through our experiences, coming into present time, and knowing ourselves, *being* ourselves as authentically as possible. During this process, we will often experience periods of doubt and confusion, sometimes even depression, as we sort through what is still real and true for us, learn to navigate by our own stars, and find our personal True North.

Engaging in this process is, of course, easier for some women than others. Many women begin to do this naturally. Some begin to write—journals, memoirs—either alone or with other women and men. Some begin to make art or scrapbooks or organize their picture albums (a very potent way of taking a trip through our past). Many take up a hobby or community project that always felt important to them but that they never felt they had time for when their days were spent tending to others' needs. They do these things naturally. They aren't even aware of the timeliness of the deeper process they are engaged in, which is essentially a life review. It is also a great time of life to find a therapist or life coach with whom you resonate—a mentor to help sift through the material, both obvious and hidden, and find the treasures.

Many women just feel lost. Often the stories we have told ourselves about the how and why of events in our lives past just don't ring true anymore. It is not as easy as it once was to hide the truth—and the knowledge of what our work is—from ourselves. I have often thought that we string memories together, like beads on a necklace, to create our history and the current image we hold of ourselves—choosing with care the memories and events that tell the stories of our lives. Then we literally tell these stories over and over again, further solidifying our present view of ourselves and offering them up as proof. We could literally go back and choose *other* stories and memories from the very same life and string them together to show quite a different history of "self" and would thereby arrive in a different present.

In the same way that holding a lighted candle to a dark window will organize the scratches into a halo with all rays pointing toward the flame, holding up a different lens to our past can reorganize our experiences and bring them to a different conclusion. We are able to separate what actually happened from the story we told ourselves about it at the time, the meaning we gave it. We arrive in a different present, a different place of consciousness, where we own those experiences as past and parts of ourselves, so that we see what is real and they no longer own us. We can see different possibilities of who we once were and are now.

Accept There Is an End

As we reach midlife, we also begin to spend more time thinking about our mortality. For some women, this brings things sharply into focus and yields unimaginable richness. For others, it brings stark terror. We have been so supported in this culture to remain "young" and to think of ourselves as perpetually youthful that many of us do not have in place any kind of belief structure or container for moving toward death. Even on our deathbeds we are not able to talk about the fact that we are dying.

When we are young, we feel immortal. Once we arrive at midlife, our parents and even many of our contemporaries may become chronically ill and begin to die around us. It takes us by surprise and so traumatizes us. The road ahead often begins to look bleak. At this point, we begin to look at life and death in a new way. We are more aware that life will end, and we begin to think about whether we have accomplished what we wanted to, lived the things that we wanted to.

Sometimes people become less afraid of death as they age because as time passes, it feels more natural for things to be drawing to a close. But sometimes this has the opposite effect. The inevitability becomes clearer and people become terrified.

The beliefs we hold about what happens when we die often shape the second half of life. If dying is something we are comfortable with, we continue to live and explore the richness of life—and we slowly prepare for our death while living each day fully. If we are in terror of it, we might shut down or focus on trying to reclaim our youth. Midlife is a time to begin to make our peace with the fact that life on earth is a journey with a beginning, a middle, and an end, and so to begin to map out what we hope to accomplish in the time remaining to us.

What is your relationship to death at the present time? Has it changed as you have aged? Are you more or less fearful? Often how we feel about death relates to how we feel about change in general. People cope with it in different ways. Think about how you usually react to big changes in your life. Aside from the general disruption they might cause, are you generally curious or excited about things changing or does it cause you to freeze up? Keep this in mind as we move forward in this exploration.

Anchor in the Present

Once we have sifted through our past, come to better know our authentic selves, and have arrived in present time, it becomes important to anchor that present self, have it witnessed, and begin to express it in the world. For a life process to be complete, we need not only to integrate our own experiences and learn from them but also to mentor others, share our wisdom, and give the gift of our lives, our learning, our authentic selves, back to the world. Ours is not a culture, like some, where a woman's status increases once her childbearing years are over and she is seen as a community treasure because of her wisdom. But it could be.

Course correction is a process that takes time and space, both physically and emotionally. It has always amazed me, for example, that our culture expects a pregnant woman to grow a new human being from scratch while still taking care of everything else she is responsible for. Pregnancy is a natural state, not an illness, but no consideration is given to women in terms of extra time, emotional space, or physical rest. Women are expected to continue at the same pace with work, taking care of home life, and their many other responsibilities while they go through this metamorphosis.

The same holds true of self-reflection and transition during midlife. Just like with a pregnancy, your hormonal shifts are literally turning you into a different being. Please give yourself the extra time, emotional space, and physical space to engage fully in this transition. Choose the things that feel most important to keep up with and let some of the others go for a while. Give yourself permission.

The Fruitful Dark

Finding oneself on the open sea of midlife, with old ways of being no longer serving, can be overwhelming. Many women find themselves lost and depressed, and they fall into what might be thought of as a dark night of the soul. Though difficult, I have always viewed these times as a portal, an initiation into the next iteration of our lives—an indication that we are ready and preparing to interface with the world at a deeper level.

In this place, we face our truest mirror, looking at where we have been so far, gathering our strength and our gifts, consolidating, and when everything else is burned away, knowing who we are. And then we step out onto a new path. In this place, we face hard truths about the world, others, and ourselves. We are in a chrysalis, being melted down to our most basic elements of soul and self. In this primordial sludge, we plant the shining seeds of our next phase and then tend them until they are strong enough to grow. Here we find again our essential self.

We are not lost, even though it feels that way. I call this "clutch time," as when you put in the clutch of a car, it allows you to move out into any gear or direction. It is a place of all possibility, and I see it as essentially hopeful, because on some level, we know we are ready to bring something deeper into the world. *Not my dark night of the soul*, you say? I am not saying it feels like this when you are in it. But, if you can remember you carry with you the seed of your essential self, and hold tight to that, the rest burns away. Initiations are hard. They are meant to be.

Later chapters will offer you some tools to use on this journey, to help you arrive in present time—authentically—in your life.

Some of these explorations will likely speak to you more than others. Each of us has different ways of knowing and experiencing the world. Some of us are more intuitive and subjective, looking to our own experiences to inform us of what is right and true and of how the world around us works. Others of us are more objective, taking in information from others, being receivers of knowledge from other sources. We look for structure from an outside source to build on. Whatever your ways of navigating, if you are ready, begin it now.

Going Deeper

Getting Our Bearings

Here are a few basic questions to begin charting your course. These questions will help you gather your tools and allies before beginning in earnest.

- Think back to the other major transitions of your life. Were you aware of them at the time, or did things only become clear once they were over?

- How did you experience these previous transitions? Were you able to give them space? Or did you feel you needed to return to or push through to what was previously known?

- What stories do you use most often to support your current view of yourself? Identify at least three.

- What tools do you usually use to navigate when you come up against the unknown? Do you research? Listen within? Talk with mentors?

- What lets you know that you have an answer that is true for you? Do you feel it somewhere in your body? Just have a sense of knowing? See it reflected in the mirroring of others?

- How can you create the space in your life to explore this major transition, menopause? Do you feel ready? If not, why not?

- Who will be your allies in this transition through midlife and menopause?

- Do you have a reliable mirror, like an old and trusted friend, who has walked the path with you, and can help to reality check you? If not, think about how you might bring this into your life.

It's important to be able to embrace change, but it is challenging for many people. Identifying how we have successfully done this before, what tools we used, and what supports we need is a good place to start. Identifying these things ahead of time is helpful because it is even more challenging when we are in the middle of change. Many of us have our plates so full that we are barely hanging on to the present, much less thinking into the future.

Thinking about our eventual death is uncomfortable for many women. If this is true for you, allow room for those feelings of discomfort and find someone you can explore this with. Think about where you might be in the transition to the Wisdom years. It is useful to identify which people, institutions, and roles you have used to navigate in your life thus far. Gather your resources, create some space, and prepare to begin.

Chapter 15

Coming into
Present Time

Tell me what you yearn for and I shall tell you who
you are. We are what we reach for, the idealized
image that drives our wandering. —James Hillman

I n earlier sections of self-inquiry, we began to sift through the
past in terms of particular areas of experience, such as early
parenting and self-concept, our sexuality, and relationships.
This investigation has helped us to see how we arrived where we are
now; what still rings true and what no longer does. Moving forward,
we will be looking at what of that still lives within us and might be
unresolved. First, though, we will turn our attention to examining
how we put many of our past experiences together to create a history and a path to how we see ourselves in present time.

It may surprise you that many of the stories you have told yourself about why you are who you are no longer ring true. If this is the
case, there is no better time than the present to rewrite them or trace
a different path of memories to a new destination—a present that is
authentic to who you know yourself to be now and that you will feel
good about taking with you into the future.

Again, if any of these explorations cause you discomfort, you
can choose to pass on by. However, there is great richness to be
found in the places we might be hesitant to enter. You might

instead choose to do that part of the exploration with a trusted friend or therapist. Sometimes it helps to have an old friend who experienced some of this with you and can mirror an alternate view to the one you see. Most of all, allow yourself time. Don't rush. In order to walk a true path into the past and not just go down the stepping-stones already in place, we need to create time for spaciousness, and have an open mind and heart.

As mentioned earlier, we all have different ways of knowing and connecting with our life experiences. For some, it may be easy to cut to the chase and find the moments in time and the experiences that have had a deep impact on us. For others, material will be much more nebulous and unconscious. I encourage you to pay attention to the feelings in your body when you think about these issues or memories. As we know, our bodies remember things our conscious minds do not. If we identify where in our body we are having feelings when we think about a particular issue, and remember another earlier time when we might have felt that way, it will often lead us back to memories and experiences that are useful in unraveling our history.

While doing these explorations, create some way to chart your path to present time—write in a journal, make art, create something with your hands to symbolize a particular moment or insight. Whatever you choose, make sure you can go back and follow the path. Enjoy the journey, and may it be a fruitful one for you.

String of Pearls

First, we will look at how our current view of ourselves came to be. What were the stories and memories that we told over and over that began to solidify as our sense of self? Is it a true view of ourselves or is it made up entirely of the voices and reflections of others? When we are very young, we create a sense of self based on the ways others respond to us. But at some point, we begin to have a sense of whether the views of others resonate with what we feel internally. Sometimes this creates a split between the internal and external. Let's first look at where our stories come from.

Using the image of beads strung on a necklace that I described earlier, choose a trait or characteristic that you feel is a core part of your identity as you see yourself now. (I am smart. I am stubborn. I am fat. I am shy. I am a person who can get things done. I am someone people can rely on.) It is most useful to choose something that you are not so happy with or a way that you view yourself that you feel holds you back. Then choose three memories or stories about yourself that you feel support that trait or characteristic.

It is helpful to choose memories from different parts of your life so that you can begin to see the path. Try choosing an early memory first. If you can remember as far back as three years old, that would be a good time—or five or six, if you can't. If you can't remember an early experience, see if you can remember a story that a parent or family member told about you at that age. Then choose a memory from your latent years (ages eight to ten) or your early teen years and one from early adulthood.

Next, see if you can look at this story as an objective observer. Try to separate out what happened, the actual sequence of events, from the story you tell about it or the meaning you ascribe to it. If it is an image you have of yourself, follow it back. Whose reflections were these—a parent, a teacher, a friend, or images from the media that you internalized? Be as completely honest as you can.

- Write down the images or stories that you chose.

- Why do you feel you chose the particular stories you did? Why are they so potent?

- If you were to sift back through your memories and experiences, what are some memories with a different flavor from the same time period that you could have chosen to create your history, but didn't? Why?

- Who would you be now if you had used this other set of moments to define yourself?

- How did these choices, or seeing yourself the way you did, serve you at the time? For example, did it help you fit in with your family? Did it feel safe?

- Does this vision of yourself accurately reflect you and serve you in the present time? If not, what are some concrete steps you can take to change this? (Sometimes it is as simple as using different memories and claiming different traits—"acting as if" you were different or a thing were true.)

Go through this process with four or five characteristics that you feel define you in ways that are no longer true (if they ever were). For each, identify whose voices or reflections highlighted this particular trait or story for you and who reinforced it. If you were the one who reinforced it, why? Sometimes knowing why can help you to separate the story from the reality.

Once you are clear about what no longer resonates, pull out the alternate memories that highlight what does feel more resonant. Replay those over and over and feel them in your body. This can be a daily meditation for a few minutes each day, until you begin to feel yourself detach from the old stories. Choose an activity or way of expression that represents the new way of seeing yourself and begin to engage in that. Gradually you will begin to inhabit present time as the version of you that you know yourself to be.

You can use this method of inquiry to look at any personality traits, reactions, characteristics, or experiences that you feel have come to define you but that no longer feel right. Don't be surprised to find that a defining moment for a point of view might have come very early in life, often before you were even talking or aware of yourself as a separate being. It is often someone else's view entirely that has been repeated down through time and taken on as personal truth.

What's Missing

If we are going to chart a course to our True North, our authentic selves, it is important to know what we feel is missing in the present. If we are going to fully inhabit ourselves, we need to feel full, have abundant inner resources to draw on, be able to easily access that inner voice that lets us know what is true for us. In order to do that, we need to identify what we feel is missing *now*, so that we can cultivate those resources.

People spend a lot of time in our culture thinking about what they don't have, never had, or missed out on. This kind of thinking holds us tethered to the past and to loss. My belief is that this attitude comes from living in a society that is based on desire—the marketing that saturates our lives and tells us that if we only had X, Y, or Z, our lives would be complete and we would be satisfied or worthy. Keeping up with the Joneses is a national pastime, and we tend to spend more time thinking about what we want and don't have than what we do have and are grateful for.

What is missing and what we desire often go hand in hand. There are desires that come from external sources (that marketing and lifestyle gurus might create) and desires (often unconscious) that stem from very early in life. Complete the statements below. The first time through, try to respond without thinking very much about it. Write down your first thought or reaction. There is usually a response there, right on the tip of your tongue. That is the one that will likely lead you back to the earliest time. You can always come back and think more about things later, but you can never recover that initial gut reaction.

- One thing I always wanted was . . .

- What I *needed* from my mother and didn't get was . . .

- What I *needed* from my father and didn't get was . . .

- One of the things I can't forgive is . . .

- If only I had (or was) _____, everything would be alright.

- What I need and never received from a man/woman is . . .

- Life would be complete if only . . .

- What I *wanted* from my mother and didn't get was . . .

- What I *wanted* from my father and didn't get was . . .

- I wouldn't have to worry if only . . .

- If only _____ hadn't happened, my life would be completely different.

- I   ise . . .

- I w   my life
  bec

- If on

- If only

- If I could change one thing, it would be . . .

- When I was young, everyone else had . . .

- What do I desire at this point in life? Do I feel I
  deserve it?

- Am I able to engage in my desires without inhibition
  or do I struggle with guilt when I want the things that
  will bring me pleasure? What do I allow to stop me?

What came up for you in this exercise? Were there any
surprises? If so, what did they tell you about your desires
and losses up until this stage of your life? It may feel overwhelming to bring up all of this material. If, for instance,
you feel a deep loss or wound around what you never
received from your mother, and your mother is no longer
living, you may wonder how you will ever begin to heal
that, learn to nurture yourself, and provide for yourself
what you find missing.

At the very least, talking about these things helps to
sort them out. Midlife is a great time to find a therapist
you trust, who can offer concrete help to move through
difficult material. You might be surprised at how just
identifying and acknowledging our losses, out loud,
opens up space for new ways of being. I would suggest
doing this exploration more than once. The first time,

write down your initial reactions. Based on what you find, take more time with the material the second time through. These things may change as you change your ways of being in the world. A journal is a good place to keep track of what begins to open up for you through these exercises.

Turning Points

It is said that whenever we choose between two paths, the one not chosen closes and is forever lost to us. While that is true in some regard, and there are choices that will forever change the course of our lives, it is possible to meander back in the direction of an earlier fork in the road. Sometimes we find ourselves back at a familiar place but with different eyes, which allow us to see the terrain in ways we couldn't before. Sometimes experiences we lacked in the first instance allow us access to what we were not wholly ready for in the past.

Some turning points in our lives make us who we are, for better or worse. Those choices might involve trauma, relationships, jobs, where we live, who we allow into or cut out of our lives. Some choices or mistakes are not possible to redo and we must live with the consequences, and for others, we are allowed a second chance.

Let's take a look at this in your life up until now. Get out your journal, a piece of paper, or drawing materials and retrace the steps of your journey. Creating a time line of important events helps you look at how the major events of your life unfolded. Make a long horizontal line on your paper, beginning at birth, and as you think of things, chart them along this time line and write down the age at which they happened.

- Can you think of some turning points that irrevocably changed your life? At what age did they occur? Who was involved?

- Were you in control or was something done to you?

- Were they related to: Relationships? Health issues? Jobs? A family matter out of your control? An action you took that you can never take back? A goal reached or not reached?

Then ask these questions:

- Why did these turning points change you?

- How did they change you?

- Would you do them over if you had a chance to?

- What choices might you make differently?

- Is there anything you can do now to take yourself closer to where you want to be in that area?

- Have you made peace with what happened or is it still very present for you?

Step back from your list and see if there is a larger question there, a pattern of some sort that you can see—for example, not putting yourself forward because you feared judgment or not allowing someone to love you because you didn't believe you deserved it. Do you believe you have the right to have what you want and choose for yourself? If you see a pattern, make a note of it.

Does making a time line and asking these questions make you aware of anything from the past that you still hold on to but that you feel you would benefit by letting go of? If we are going to live in the present, we must look at our past and see what needs to be celebrated and mourned from each stage of life that came before. For example, a woman may have had an abortion in the past, or made a choice to move down the path of career rather than having a child, and find herself at menopause grieving that choice. She no longer *has* the option to have a biological child and needs to find a way to make peace with that. This can be hard, but she can give herself time and space to grieve this, celebrate the gifts her choice brought to her, and then go about finding other ways to have children or mentees in her life in a way that allows her to experience some of what she missed by not being a mother.

Once you have identified repeated past patterns, it will be important to keep these in the forefront of your mind going forward, so that you don't continue to repeat them. Identify small steps you can take right now to bring yourself back toward where you would like to be.

If you had to give up a cherished dream of a certain job or career because of childbearing and childrearing, perhaps you could now go back to school and slowly pick up courses that will lead you toward that goal or give you the joy of learning. If you took a path that led you away from family and you would like to repair that, reach out. Once we acknowledge this material and stop hiding from it, the way forward becomes easier to see. We want to arrive in the present as free of baggage as possible while honoring our authentic self.

Hide and Seek

It's the unconscious things that often throw us off center the most. We don't see their influence because they are hidden, and therefore we cannot make allies of them. How do we begin to think about what we are hiding from ourselves or what is hiding from us? These things are hidden, after all, and probably for a reason. However, there is usually a persistent nudge in our lives from these things. They keep reminding us they are there. They are waiting for us to be ready to receive them.

I have always been interested in what makes a moment of change possible when it wasn't before. What brings us to a point where we can lift up our foot and put it down into a new world? Sometimes it is having cultivated a new perspective, or having experienced something that lets us know our true strength or allowed us to grow empathy for another. Sometimes it is just having reached a certain age or a certain knowledge that we *must* express ourselves, regardless of whether we fit into the cultural narrative or meet the expectations of others. When women reach menopause, what I often hear is "If not now, when?" You will be much more prepared now to face a moment of change—and have more courage to do so—having completed previous explorations that looked at all the things that have brought you to this moment in life.

Here are some questions to get you started in looking for what is hidden in your life. You may think of others. Take some time with these. Because of their nature, the answers may not be at the tip of your tongue, and you may have to meditate on them or let them bubble up at their own pace. Answers may come to you in a dream or when you are engaged in tasks that allow your mind to wander.

I would encourage you to set aside time as you begin to consider each one. Think of the question consciously. Write down any thoughts that immediately come to mind and then leave some space to go back and add things that will show themselves over time. If you feel any of this might bring up material that would be difficult to handle alone, please engage the help of a friend or therapist to be your touchstone.

What am I afraid to know? These may be things that circle back into your consciousness over and over. It may be a thought or a period of time you keep coming back to, or a memory—because you know it is important—but there is the feeling that if you *really* let it come, you would have to change your life and the way you see yourself and others see you in the world. It becomes easier to just leave it alone. Sometimes we screen the real memory with a similar "memory," yet when we think about it, something doesn't feel quite right.

There may also be a feeling that this time period holds a lot of your energy prisoner, so that it is not available to you. If you face the fear in what you are afraid to know and bring it into the light of consciousness, the trapped energy will be released, so that you can use it. You need to be ready to do this, however.

What do I ALMOST know? In the same way that a memory might not feel quite right, thoughts and perspectives can also feel not quite right. We may have spent a lifetime with certain beliefs and been very comfortable speaking and living them, and then at some point, they don't quite ring true anymore. The minute the words leave our mouth, we know they are not really true for us now. But we don't have anything yet to replace them with, so we continue to live as if they do, saying the same things and telling the same stories. If this is true for you, just write down what you become aware of and allow it to percolate. What might happen if you opened to embrace something different? Is there a fear there, or have you just not taken the time to see how things have changed?

What knowledge am I avoiding, even though I know it is important? This might have to do with lifestyle or health issues, something you need to address but don't feel you have the time or emotional bandwidth to tackle yet. It may have to do with a friendship or intimate relationship that is not working anymore, or a job you have lost all energy for. Take an honest look, even if you are not yet ready to share that knowledge with anyone yet, or—if you are ready—take steps to change it. Knowing is an important first step.

What am I consciously hiding—from myself, from others? There often comes a point in the process of change where we have become clear within ourselves what needs to change but we are not ready to be public with it yet. This is a signpost on the road of becoming more authentic. It is important to make the distinction between what we know but are not ready to share and what we don't know or *almost* know. We can first begin to anchor that in ourselves, "try it on" before we step into the expression of it.

Women are *very* intuitive about what is true and real. We know deep down when we are avoiding something or when something doesn't ring true. Protecting ourselves from this allows us to engage in "business as usual" and not disrupt our lives, but it also holds us back. It is important to tell ourselves the truth, even if we are not ready to share it yet.

The Best-Laid Plans . . .

Menopause is a perfect time to check in with our life plans and make new ones, if we want to. Most of us carry with us a vague (or maybe specific) idea of where we wanted to be at this stage of our lives. This can be centered around career, an intimate partner, children, or finances. We may have gauged this against our parents, siblings, or a mentor in our lives. Sometimes feelings of failure can ensue if we are not where we had hoped to be. This can relate to some of our "forks in the road" and the choices we made. However, it is very useful to look at where we find ourselves now in relationship to the dreams and plans we made in our younger years to see if they are even true for us anymore.

These answers will come easily for most people. Get out your journal or a piece of paper and look at where you are in relationship to your goals around the following things:

Finances

- Do you have the level of income you hoped for at this time of life? Is it enough to meet your needs? If not, how does that make you feel?

- Have you prepared for retirement? Have you met goals you had, to be able to spend the last arc of your life in the manner you wish to? Maybe you have never considered that retirement is an option for you. If this is the case, look at how you might shift the work you do to be more suited to this last phase of life.

- Do you feel you are being paid commensurate with what you are providing in your work?

- Do you feel you have the knowledge you need to navigate the financial part of your life going forward?

- Is there someone (family, friends, coworkers) who you judge yourself by or feel competitive with? If so, who? Why?

- Have you made a will or done any estate planning you wish to do?

Relationships

- If you were to have an injury, illness, or devastating emotional loss, do you have a support system in place?

- Do you have an intimate partner? Was this a goal for you? Is it okay if you don't?

- Do you have children, grandchildren? Was this a strong desire for you?

- Is there a larger community you feel a part of?

Work in the World

- Did you embark on a career or have you chosen different kinds of work as your life unfolded, and are you where you hoped you would be on that path?

- Does the work you chose to do still nourish you or has it lost its meaning?

- Do you feel you have been adequately recognized for the work you do?

- Are you happy to stick with the work/career you chose and are engaged in at the present time or is there something else you would like to do with the remaining arc of your life?

- If you could be doing anything you want at this time of your life, what would it be?

Once you have finished, take a look at what you have written. Are you generally on track with your life plans? Had you been aware of them specifically or did you just have a vague sense of where you wanted to be? Looking at this, how does it make you feel?

Don't be discouraged if you are not where you want to be. Remember, "you can pull any thread and unravel the Universe." It is not a long trip from "here" to "there," from A to B. You are always on the path. Just start where you are and take a step, a true step. If each step you take is a true step, you will end up in the right place. Every step also has a ripple effect. You may find yourself in a very different place before you know it.

Taking Stock

Now that you have taken a good long look at your past and what brought you to present time, it is important to take stock of where you are and pull it together. Where do you stand now in relationship to your life plans? What did you find out? Are you where you thought you would be at this point in your life? What tools do you have to make change? What are your successes, overall? Where have you not lived up to your own expectations or those of others? Does it matter? Are those goals still relevant?

At midlife, we benefit from looking at whether we are still waiting to live our lives. Some questions to ponder are:

- Do you spend your time at something you love or do you do what must be done in order to get by, make ends meet, and dream of the "someday" when you can live your life as you choose?

- Do you spend your time in a way that is meaningful to you and compatible with your ethics and values or do you need to set those aside in order to make a living?

- Are you spending time with people who you respect and consider friends and allies?

- Do you have people in your life with whom you can be completely yourself, who you feel really know you? Who are they?

It is also important, as we enter into this next phase and begin to do the integration work, to look at what we might consider our spiritual selves, or our consciousness. Some questions to contemplate:

- Do you have a sense of purpose in your life?

- Do you have a sense of why you are here on Earth?

- Does your life have meaning?

- Do you feel you are fulfilling your potential? What are you proud of? What are your regrets?

How able we feel to create what we want and go after it is also important if we are going to bring it into reality for ourselves. Therefore, it is useful to ask:

- What is your relationship to desire? Do you allow it, work toward fulfilling it?

- Does wanting something make you feel guilty, selfish? This is often the case for women.

- What can you add to your life right now that will nourish you?

Our sense of what is possible is critical here. Many of us have led lives that allow us to feel that we have the tools, skills, and the right to go after what we want in the world. Many of us have not led our lives in this way, or even if we have, we feel trapped in our current circumstances because of commitments or responsibilities that demand we stay where we are for the income it brings. Here are some questions to help you look at where you stand in relationship to possibility in your life:

- Do you feel like you have options in regard to the important matters in your life or do you feel trapped in an experience you can't get out of?

- What is your sense of your future? Do you feel generally optimistic, pessimistic, or resigned?

- Do you feel safe?

- How do you feel about the state of the world? Do you feel that you have any power to affect what you see?

- What will it take for you to take the next step in your life and move toward a future that allows you to live authentically?

- Is change easier or more difficult for you as you age?

These are just some of the questions you can explore to help you assess where you are right now. Here are a few general questions that you can engage with as well, if you feel drawn to, and *tell yourself the truth* as you know it—no hiding from yourself or "looking good." If you want this exercise to be most useful, you need to be honest and do the work.

What is working:

- What do you feel you are doing right?

- What have you accomplished that you set out to do? If not, why not?

- What are your "deal-breakers"? Are you honoring them?

- Do you know how to say no? Yes?

Taking stock is a big piece of work. It can bring up many feelings in us and sometimes a sense of anxiety as well. I recommend that you sit with this information for a little while after completing this exploration. Let things settle in and begin to bubble up. Don't make judgments about yourself or circumstances too quickly. And most of all, give yourself a little time before making changes.

Stepping into the Future

Stepping into the future involves making some choices and being ready to advocate for your own life rather than simply being the support system for other people's dreams at the expense of your own. We are essentially tribal animals. When people step outside of cultural norms, there are consequences. This can have both positive and negative aspects to it.

Begin by listing ten things that you currently spend your time and life force doing every day, *instead* of what you feel you really *should* be spending it on or what you *want* to be spending it on. Then see how you feel about the questions below. Looking at this last set of questions will tell you a lot about your chosen road ahead, what you feel you need to prioritize to feel good about where you are in your life and to not leave a great weight of the "undone" behind you when your life comes to a close.

Integration—taking all the knowledge we have accumulated and making some sense of it—is the developmental task in this last arc of our lives.

Consider:

- Are you paying enough attention to what is going on around you?

- Do you care too much about what people think of you? Does this restrict your choices? (*What will people think?* Many women in my generation were raised with this being paramount.)

- Have you forgiven those you need to?

- How do you want to be remembered? What legacy do you want to leave?

- Have you created succession—that is, passed on what you know to someone coming behind you? Have you mentored anyone?

- Have you made your peace with the fact that you are a mortal being and will die someday?

- What is your role in the community you live in?

- What is still undone that you want to accomplish before you die? What is one step you can take now toward that goal?

Your Perfect World

As we compose this next phase of our lives, it can be useful to dream into our perfect world. If we could have it any way we want, how would it be? How would our day unfold? When would we awaken? With whom? What would we be doing? Where would it be? Would it be alone or with other people?

Answer these questions as if you can have anything you want, as if nothing can stand in your way. Then put your wish list up somewhere where you can see it. Begin by making any small adjustments you can make in your daily life to better align with your "perfect world." This might be something as simple as adding an hour of alone time in the morning. Some things you will not be able to change now, but as decisions and choices are made later, if you choose at each juncture to align yourself with the vision of your life as you would like to live it, you will come closer and closer to having it be the way that feels most like you.

There may be other questions or issues that rise to the surface as you begin to sift through your past. Write them down. Embrace them.

The Menopause Ritual

Once you sense you have arrived in present time, I feel it is very useful to mark this doorway into the next part of your life with ceremony. All through our lives, we participate in ceremonies to mark our passages so that friends and family can share in our happiness or grief and so that our community can support a new role for us within our tribe.

In our culture, stepping through the doorway to elderhood is not a passage that has generally been celebrated. We tend to infantilize our elders in this culture. We generally put our elders away rather than cherish them and their life wisdom. With our focus on youth, it is expected that we will retire at a certain age and trundle off to play shuffleboard in the sun for the rest of our lives and not bother the young folk as they go about ordering the world—and this at a time when many women and men are at their most potent in terms of the wisdom and life experience they have to share. Our elder years, or Wisdom years, can be ones of immense productivity and creativity, which you will see in the wonderful examples in the next section of this book.

Many women choose to mark this point in their lives with ritual. Having taken a bold look at their lives and acknowledged an authentic self in the making, they wish to make a commitment to this self in the presence of their community. These menopause rituals, or "cronings," that women create are as individual as they are, but to my mind, they should contain four elements: an acknowledgment of what is being left behind, an acknowledgment of what is being brought forward, and commitments or vows to what the next phase of life will be dedicated to—and this should all be done in the presence of witnesses. Witnessing is an active and very important piece of speaking our truth into the world—until it is received, it is not activated.

For my own menopause ritual, I chose to gather with about seven close women friends and take them on a journey through my life. I had moved to my present community in my midforties, become a new mother here, and entered into a role and lifestyle that was much different from what my earlier years had been about. Consequently I felt that my community didn't know the whole me—just the slice that was the mother.

I got out my box of photographs, and beginning with pictures of my parents, I showed my friends where I came from. I briefly took them through my early life, my girlhood dreams, my years in theater and delivering babies, my important relationships, my two marriages—and I illustrated all of this with pictures. We discussed the turning points I had become aware of and where I had submerged my own voice in order to support others. Step by step we trod the path to present time. From that place I then made my vows in front of them to the second half of my life. I made promises as to what I would dedicate my energy to, the level of truth I would try to live within, and I asked them all to hold me accountable to this. There was, of course, also lots of good food, music, and dancing!

Other menopause rituals I have heard of, or have participated in, were like big parties, with a piece of time taken out in the middle for the woman to acknowledge the door she was walking through and sometimes to ask for support. One woman created a piece of art with her vows written on it and then had everyone present sign it in support. This is framed and hanging in her home now as a permanent reminder of the promises she made and the women who hold her accountable to those promises. Another woman I know gathered a group of women over a weekend and created a beautiful ceremonial robe, which hangs in her home and which she will wear on special occasions. And yet another chose to share her goals and commitments to the next phase of her life and then have every woman there offer her their wisdom to take with her on that journey. The possibilities are as numerous and diverse as we are.

There is something very precious about declaring oneself and being fully seen. It liberates a tremendous amount of energy, which is usually used to keep up the social façade. Once this energy is liberated, the possibilities grow exponentially.

Here is a template to use, if you wish, to create your ritual.

1. Think about how you generally express yourself. Are you visual? Intellectual? Kinesthetic? Do you tell stories often? You will be marking an important passage. What sort of activity will give this the most meaning and express who you are at your core?

2. Begin to think about your life to this point. Did you end up where you thought you would? If not, why not—and is this a positive or a negative thing? Use the self-inquiry you have done to this point to begin to sift through losses, disappointments, accomplishments, and surprises (both positive and negative).

3. With whom would you feel comfortable sharing this information? If you want to keep the fruits of your introspection private and just share a "stepping through" ritual of some kind, or have a party, that is fine. Be aware, though, that having witnesses to these things

helps us to solidify and release them. It also allows us to ask for support from our community for expressing our authenticity.

4. Decide how you want to mark this transition and who you want to be with you when you do.

5. Decide what you want to commit your life energy to for the remainder of your life.

6. Gather your materials (photos, music, journals, gifts for those who will be there, etc.).

7. Make your invitations. This can be a very creative part of the ritual, and the energy that goes into making them begins the ritual. It also honors the ones you choose to share this with.

8. Show up. Have fun. Laugh, cry, take in the love of those who show up for you.

9. Take steps to put in place what you will need to begin your new commitments.

Express yourself!

This chapter has likely brought up a huge amount of material for digesting. There might have been a few surprises and possibly a significant shift in perspective that will take time to integrate. I hope you have given yourself the time to go through it slowly and really finish with each exercise before moving on. Take the opportunity to allow things to bubble up over time before jumping to take action. Give yourself that time. If you find yourself drawn back to a particular exercise, think about why. Maybe do it again when you are ready and see if you can go deeper this time.

What is most important to keep in mind is that you are moving toward a place of authenticity, what is most authentic to you *now*. You are distilling the Wise Woman within you, mixing the brew of your life experience and distilling the potent essence. This is a process, not an exercise you do once and move on. Finding home and your True North is an evolving journey.

Chapter 16

Becoming the Wise Woman

Who is the crone? She is the most dangerous, the most radical, the most revolutionary woman in existence. Whether in fairy tales or in consensual reality, the old one goes where she wants to and she acts as she wishes; she lives as she chooses. And this is all as it should be. And no one can stop her. Nor ought they try. —Clarissa Pinkola Estés

After completing the journey of the previous chapter with depth, attention, and time, you will have arrived more caught up to present time and aware of the scaffolding that supports your sense of self. Your feelings may be close to the surface. Even if there is material you haven't been able to shift that you would like to, you are now more aware of it and therefore it does not drive your behavior in such an unconscious way.

Also, after sifting through much of your past material, you have made some choices about what still resonates as true. You may have made some commitments to the next phase of your life in front of witnesses who will hold you accountable. I sometimes jokingly think of it as preparing for the Yard Sale of Life, in that we pick up each memory, experience, assumption, and judgment, look it over and remember how it came to us, assess whether we still have use for it, check to see if it still reflects us, and then decide whether to get rid of or keep it. Along the way, especially if sharing the process with friends, we shed a tear or two, have a good belly laugh, and probably even dance around the room a bit! When something does not ring true, we are aware of it—even as we hear the words leave our mouths. We can no longer hide from ourselves, nor do we desire to.

You should be much closer now to being fully present in your life through menopause and beyond, aware of what your truth is, and what your authentic stance is in the world. As you feel into the future from here, questions arise, and there are decisions to be made. Does the way you conduct your life reflect your authentic self? Do your friendships, your current relationships, your job reflect who you want to be in the world as an elder woman? It is useful sometimes to do another permutation of the "good for me/ bad for me" list you made earlier while evaluating the stress in your life, except now it would read more like an authentic/not authentic list, as you turn a bold eye to how you wish to spend your life force.

You may feel that there are things about your life that no longer reflect you, yet not have a clear sense about what it would look like to live in a way that does. I would encourage you to think back to when you were ten or eleven years old, before the hormone tidal wave hit, and remember what your dreams were then. What called to you? What did you feel passionate about? We are often very clear at that age about who we are and what we are to be in the world.

I remember giving my daughter a tape recorder when she was in the fifth grade and encouraging her to talk to her future self. She seemed so very clear then, and I knew what was coming when the hormones hit. We are thrown under and tumbled by the force of that wave and don't come up for many years. By then, we have often forgotten the clarity of our girl years. We do, in fact, come with operating instructions; we just can't find them in any book. They reside in the cells of our body, in our DNA, and we must feel into them, live into them, in order to receive the wisdom they have to impart to us.

Pay attention also to your nighttime dreams. This is a great time to start a dream journal, make a wish map, get out the pastels and paper and draw the images that come through. Our dreams can be very clear way-showers.

Don't be surprised if you find that there is a split between the inner and outer material—the images and activities of your dream life and that of your day-to-day life. This is entirely normal. What you are doing is creating a pathway for your inner voice to communicate with you. It is sometimes the way our body tells us what it knows, that we haven't seen before. Once the pathway is established, it will yield a wealth of information. This is important work. Carl Jung once said, "The greater the disparity between the outer and inner person, the greater the chance for trouble."

Even if this process seems difficult, you can still move forward. Sometimes all you need to know is the first step, or just to feel an impulse. At the very least, before just reacting to something, you can take a beat and ask yourself, *What do I really think about this?*

My client Christine remembered how much she enjoyed baking with her grandmother when she was a little girl. She had spent her adult life as a busy attorney, which gave her no free time to indulge in anything else. As a result of doing a midlife inventory, she realized she had spent a life pursuing a job that made her parents happy but no longer reflected her authentic self in the world. She wasn't sure she could give it up, however, because she had made commitments to certain schooling for her kids and to a lifestyle she had created with her family. She did commit, though, to doing something to bring more pleasure into her life, and what she chose was to carve out some time to bake on weekends. She loved it so much that she parlayed it into a cupcake business that is doing very well. She is happy, less stressed, and enjoying her life.

We are stepping into the role of Wise Woman, both personally and culturally. We are integrating our experience, owning our wisdom. Our next step is to pass that on. We can live a bright flare of a life, but it dies with us if we have not created succession—if we have not mentored others to take our place, learn from our experience, and make it their own. The world desperately needs the wisdom of women at this juncture. We are born with the tools to give birth, nurture, raise up, even if we do not choose to literally do these things. The Wise Woman is a very powerful archetype, and in ancient times it was revered. What does that mean for us?

When the Hag Enters, the Story Changes

The function of the crone, or the Wise Woman, in stories and especially in fairy tales is that of the magician (or witch), the shapeshifter, the knower of the ways of the Earth. When she appears in a story, you know the transformation is about to begin for the Traveler, or the protagonist. She shows the Traveler parts of themselves that they didn't know existed; she holds up the mirror of truth. She gives the gift of magic beans, sets the tasks that will transform the Traveler into their realized self.

The words *crone* and *hag* have taken on negative or ugly connotations in our patriarchal times, but when the words were first coined, in a time when the Great Goddess ruled over all of the passages of our lives—the births, the bloodings, the marriages, and the deaths—she was known for what she is. The word *crone* comes from *crown*, and indicates wisdom emanating from the head. The word *hag* comes from *hagio*, meaning holy.

In modern times, the crone has morphed more into the ageless Wisdom goddess, the Wise Woman, but the characteristics are the same. She looks at life with a bold eye, does not hide from the truth, and impartially sees what others fail to see. At this point in our lives, we are generally more free to concentrate on ourselves, to pan for the gold in the river that our life has been and be fully capable, fully sexual, and regarded as independent agents in our communities. We can *compose* a life, not be a victim to it or just follow along with someone else's script.

Wise Women don't hide. They take full responsibility for themselves and generally care a lot less about what people think than they did at earlier times in life. This is one of the great gifts of menopause that I have seen emerge over and over, both in my own life and that of other women. We just don't spend as much time thinking about what other people will think of our choices or actions. We don't let that determine whether we tell a truth or do a deed. Not to say we run rampant in the face of our community's values, but we don't give truth to the lie.

There is also a phenomenon happening more these days as women enter the workforce in greater numbers and choose not to have children, where a woman essentially passes from being a maiden to a crone without ever being a mother or a matron. Even among those women who have chosen to have children, we tend to be youthful longer, stay active, and segue straight from our youth to our elder years, essentially bypassing middle age. Does skipping this step make our arrival at our elder years more jarring? More of a surprise? Are we missing out on a whole phase of life and the life tasks that go with it? It is interesting to contemplate.

Not all women become Wise Women, nor wish to. Being a Wise Woman is not something that automatically comes with having reached a certain age or stage in life. It is a conscious acceptance of responsibility for your own life and actions, of being responsible to your truth and authenticity and giving that back to the world. The Wise Woman knows that she is the composer of her own life and does not merely live the script that is handed to her. It is not something to be taken on lightly, but I believe it is part of Nature's intention for us, and the rewards are great if we do, for ourselves and our communities.

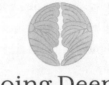

Going Deeper

Exploring the Wise Woman
Archetype in Your Life

It is important to take a minute or two to stop and think about what our younger selves imagined this time of life would be like—if we thought about it at all. The truth is more often that when we are young, we can't really imagine ourselves as aging. It is sometimes hard to imagine aging even when we are right in the middle of it. However, our images and intentions set a template of sorts and this can be either positive or negative. When we played our "perfect world" game, we put our goals and intentions in a place we could see them, framing our choices going forward. Our unconscious images and choices about where we are heading are equally as powerful. See which questions draw you, but take a look also at what you avoid. These questions often indicate what is still unconscious and hold the most juice.

- Was there an elder woman in your life as a child with whom you spent time or who you looked up to? A grandmother? A family friend? A public figure?

- Was the view of elderhood in your young world generally positive or negative?

- What qualities did you start to associate with aging—infirmity, limitation, irritability, kindness, nurturing, the ability to see what others didn't?

- How did this frame the way you thought about how you might be as an elder woman?

- When did it first hit you that you were aging? What were the first signs? Were they physical or emotional? Were they welcome? Were they scary?

- How do you see yourself functioning as an elder woman? How will it change you? How will your life be affected? Has this process already started?

- What do you fear about "old age"?

- What do you feel you will be able to celebrate about it?

- What steps can you take now to alter your path toward a positive outcome?

- What support systems do you have in place?

Being the Wise Woman doesn't mean we need to become "old." It is more about owning ourselves—that is, gathering our energies and previous identities into one coherent whole and standing in our power. Once we gather ourselves into the present, we are a force for grounding, perspective, and continuity. We see the path behind us and the possibilities for the future. We have the presence and the insight to be able to mentor those who come after us. We become evolutionary change agents. This is true whether we take on a new arc of work in the world or focus our wisdom on giving to our family. There is no right or wrong here. Once you are caught up to present time, you will know what is right for you and can step out onto your path with confidence.

PART FOUR

Moving Through

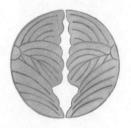

Chapter 17

Engaging and Sharing Your Wisdom

Aging is inevitable, but getting "old"
is entirely optional! —Lisa Levine

Embodying the Wise Woman, or the elder, may be the most meaningful phase of our lives, yet you wouldn't know it to scan the popular culture. Our images of aging are of loss—loss of beauty, value, energy, intelligence. So many women buy that message and just give up and begin to fade away. So much wisdom is lost in these cases, and we need it. It begs the question: Is wisdom truly wisdom if it is not shared?

Anthropologists and social biologists tell us that what actually began to move culture forward historically was women who lived past their reproductive years and had reached the age of grand-mothers. This is affectionately known as the *grandmother hypothesis*. Once we began to live past our childbearing years, we were able to serve a role that we hadn't been able to previously. We moved our evolution forward.

Women who survived long enough to become grandmoth-ers gathered more food than the men or the reproductive-aged women, and that increase in nutrition also increased brain size and longevity. Given that humans cannot fend for themselves as infants the way other species do, having a mother or adult to care for, feed, and protect an infant was very important in terms of our survival. A mother would care for a child until the next baby was born, and then the child's chances of survival would diminish as the mother's attention turned toward the new infant. With a grandmother around, the first child would continue to be nurtured, fed, and taught, both ensuring that child's survival and enabling the mother to have more children who grew to adulthood and passed on their genes.

Grandmothers also had the time and patience to teach children and, one would assume, to contemplate the spiritual nature of life—to contemplate beyond just survival—thereby waking up a totally different part of the human brain. They had a longer view and became the keepers of the larger story of their culture.

Grandmothers kept the stories and oral histories of the tribes. As time went on, in many tribal societies, the grandmothers actually became the last word on many of the tribe's activities. In many Native American tribes, it was the Council of Grandmothers who traditionally decided whether the tribe would go to war and who would marry whom, and they adjudicated many of the disputes that inevitably arose in a tribal living situation. They held a very respected place in the life of the tribe, and this was totally appropriate to their stage in life.

Many of us have stories to tell about how wonderful our own grandmothers were and how special they made us feel. The love and acceptance they brought, and the perspective and wisdom of those who had lived full lives, helped us to see further down the road to what the longer arc of a life might be than what we were able to glean from our mothers, who were often overwhelmed and barely able to see past getting food on the table at night. I know my grandmother had patience. She had time. She had resilience. She listened. She really took the time to see me. We had conversations that helped me understand humans better.

It is interesting that in the only other mammalian species who continue to live past their reproductive years, orcas and pilot whales, the role of the post-reproductive females is similar. They become the pod leaders. They help the pod survive when food sources are low, because they carry the knowledge of food resources back in time and are able to guide the pod to hunting grounds that the younger whales do not know about. Their long memories serve their community and their "grandwhales," increasing survival in the pod.

What's Next

At this point in this book's journey, you should have a much clearer view about who you are right now: what moves you, interests you, beckons to you. What did you make your commitments to during your menopause ritual? It is time to move toward that and begin to share your wisdom with others.

Sharing wisdom can come in many forms. It doesn't have to be public, if you are someone with a more introverted nature. You might choose to do as the grandmothers of old did and share your wisdom and insight within your own tribe, your family, to enrich the lives of your children and grandchildren. Some women may want to move out into their communities and volunteer—serve at a food bank or community-run clinic, hold babies in withdrawal from drugs at a local hospital, bring their problem-solving abilities to bear on local issues, run for office—to share their wisdom with the people with whom they live.

Menopausal women are uniquely suited for this. I think of Hazel McCallion, who channeled her Wisdom energy into running a city. At the age of fifty-seven, the year after her husband of twenty-seven years passed away, she was elected the first mayor of Mississauga, Ontario, Canada. She kept this job until she retired in 2014 at the age of ninety-five. Under her leadership, Mississauga became the third largest city in Ontario and the sixth largest city in Canada. During that time, the city was never in debt, and at the time of her resignation, the city had $700 million in cash reserves. She didn't campaign or accept campaign contributions, but she would instead ask constituents to give to their favorite charity. She belonged to no party and as an independent agent was able to run the city as she saw fit, since she was not beholden to a party plank. This is an elder in action.

Hazel led through transparency, inspiration, and commitment to her constituency, and by being tough, resilient, and healthy. All of these are Wise Woman attributes. She was so well loved that she ran against sixteen other candidates for her last term in office and still garnered 76 percent of the votes. She had close to a 90 percent approval rating when she retired.

Hazel didn't stop there. Three months after she retired from being mayor of Mississauga, she took a job at the University of Toronto Mississauga, where she assisted in developing a master's degree program in urban innovation and development. She continues creating and mentoring to this day.

Other women will follow their muse and develop a talent or interest from earlier in life, such as writing, painting, dancing, singing, or acting, and express themselves through these mediums. Others may go back to school, get the degree that they delayed in order to raise their children, and go out into the workforce for the first time, doing work that fulfills them.

Women already doing public work in the world often find that they have additional energy freed up for their work once the children are grown. As their hormones of creativity rise, they do some of their most potent work during these years.

Female baby boomers, a huge demographic, are reaching their Wisdom years now, and I find this very exciting. I can't think of anything this world would benefit from more than a tidal wave of elder women's energy and wisdom. However, as a generation, we have had few real models for what this can look like. This is one reason the messages of loss from the media are so easily absorbed. The women who have blazed the trails ahead of us have not readily been seen, though this has changed some in recent years.

It's Never Too Late

"It's never too late to begin; it's never too early to start."

I remember when these words from Dr. Valerie Hunt first really "landed" for me. I was in my late forties and attending a conference on prenatal life and consciousness. I experienced Dr. Hunt when she was ninety years of age and giving her last public lecture. She was speaking about the development of her latest invention and her ongoing research into the field of bioenergetics and disease.

Dr. Hunt was a scientist, an author, and a former professor of physiological science at UCLA. She did pioneering research in the field of human bioenergy, physiology, and bioengineering well into her late eighties and early nineties. At the conference, she was talking about her latest invention, which reads the bioenergetic field of the human body and can detect disruptions in this field, alerting someone to the imbalances that precede disease. Her life work has led to the scientific understanding of the relationship between energy field disturbances, disease, and emotional pathologies. I was so impressed with her vitality, clarity, and *enthusiasm* this late into her life. At ninety, she was still following her curiosity and contributing to her field. I was officially inspired.

The stories of women who just keep living their lives—living them fully—after menopause are endless. I am sure you know women in your own community to whom you could point. One thing to notice about these women: they don't recognize that they are *supposed* to fade away. We don't have to do something "big" or noticeable, as these women have. The key component to a Wisdom life is showing up, being present and authentic, and giving back in some way, sharing what you have learned.

Going Deeper

Where from Here?

Here are some things to think about as you move toward a new or added focus:

- What do you find you value the most as you age? Has this changed from your younger years? In what ways?

- Who would you want to share these things with? Toward what end?

- Does thinking about sharing your wisdom bring excitement? Fear? Confusion?

- What opportunities do you have to move toward this thing that draws you?

- What would be a first step?

- What would it take to begin something new?

- What are you willing to detach from now that you weren't willing to even a year or two ago? Why?

- What do you find you are willing to claim now that you weren't willing to a year or two ago? What happened to make this change possible?

- Who are some of the postmenopausal women in your own life who have inspired you? Why?

You should now be more caught up to present time and have released much of the old "stuff" that is using energy, even when you are not engaging with it. (Think of a tab on your computer that remains open, and even if you are not interacting with it, it uses considerable energy.) What will you do with this newly freed-up energy? You still have a very potent arc of your life to live. There are so many causes clamoring for our attention these days. So many needs to fill.

Notice what came up for you and what really drew you forward in your investigations. It may be a need you see in your community, a cause that feels particularly urgent right now. Perhaps there is something you have always wanted to do but you felt you never had the time for, an inquiry that your life has moved you toward. You are also more aware of what your gifts and your boundaries are. Make a choice for what makes you feel most alive.

Chapter 16

Becoming the
Memory Keeper

Becoming a grandmother is wonderful. One
moment you're just a mother. The next you
are all-wise and prehistoric.   —Pam Brown

We in our fifties and sixties are the last of the generations to grow up in the world before the digital age,
where life came to be lived on devices connected to
the internet. We were actual persons and interacted with people,
not their accounts. Social influence was largely carried out in person and in communities, not on Instagram. Still, ad agencies and
television had an ever-increasing influence over our desires and the
ways that we thought of ourselves as a culture. We still lived in an
analog world.

This analog world was in many ways more limited in scope
than what is offered today. However, it also contained great benefits. Life was slower, and we were not expected to be "on" and
available to everyone 24/7. We were more connected to our
communities.

We had time to let things soak in, contemplate, linger, reca-
librate, and rest. Therefore, our brains were able to engage with
many aspects of our environment that we, sped up today, no long
have the bandwidth for. Because of the pace of life, we had the last

Chapter 18

Becoming the
Memory Keeper

Becoming a grandmother is wonderful. One
moment you're just a mother. The next you
are all-wise and prehistoric.   —Pam Brown

W e in our fifties and sixties are the last of the generations to grow up in the world before the digital age,
where life came to be lived on devices connected to
the internet. We wrote actual letters and interacted with people,
not their accounts. Social influence was largely carried out in person and in communities, not on Instagram. While ad agencies and
television had an ever-increasing influence over our desires and the
ways that we thought of ourselves as a culture, we still lived in an
analog world.

This analog world was, in many ways, more limited in scope
than what is offered today. However, it also conferred great benefits. Life was slower, and we were not expected to be "on" and
available to everyone 24/7. We were more connected to our
communities.

We had time to let things soak in, contemplate, integrate, reca-
librate, and rest. Therefore, our brains were able to engage with
many aspects of our environment that we just can't today, or don't
have the bandwidth for, because of the pace of life and the fact that

we are living more virtually. We were more directly connected with Nature and therefore more grounded to Earth, to a sense of place.

Our bodies generally had a lower level of background stress as well. There was not nearly the incidence of autoimmune disease. Depression and anxiety have risen sharply over the last fifty years, particularly in teens and young adults. And even though our world has expanded greatly through the degree to which we are living virtually these days, there is much information that we *don't* have access to when we interact with someone on a screen or through an account, and we are poorer for that.

The internet alone has connected us to one another in ways and across distances that were not dreamed of even when I was well into my forties. We can now collaborate with people across the globe that we will never meet in person. This is miraculous. However, it clearly has its downside as well. As a culture, we now place most of our focus in a virtual world where a very few entities curate what information we see and how we see it and strongly flavor what we consider to be reality, despite what we see around us when we open our eyes or speak directly to one another. If something is repeated a few times and is seen in print, it becomes true, whether it is or not.

We are encouraged to identify with certain brands and people, and to be loyal to them above all else, even above what we see happening around us. We live online a kind of fantasy lifestyle that is largely unattainable in our analog world. To my mind, the situation has gone beyond the internet hugely influencing our world and the way we see it—and one another—to having created two separate but *parallel* worlds, the virtual and the analog. Even in the virtual world, there are many parallel worlds we inhabit.

The pervasive nature of our electronic devices is affecting us physically, socially, and environmentally. Children are three times more likely to be obese now than they were a generation ago, and while this is not entirely due to device addiction, the sedentary nature of this activity certainly contributes. Back in my generation, we watched some television and had Saturday morning cartoons, but they were not available twenty-four hours a day, and we spent considerable time outdoors playing and being active.

Also, our bodies now marinate in the electromagnetic field that Wi-Fi generates, and this is only becoming stronger and more pervasive. Research on how these radiation fields affect the body is still somewhat controversial, and some hasn't even been done because the corporations involved would prefer to keep it under the radar. However, there is evidence that it affects everything from mood, sleep, and our ability to concentrate to creating tissue damage, tumor and cancer development, loss of fertility, and birth defects.

Socially, we have become less present. It is not at all unusual to be out to dinner and see a couple or even a group of diners at a nearby table, each with their head in their own phone, scrolling through social media and not interacting with each other at all. They are not present to their surroundings. This most distresses me when I see a small child trying to get their parent's attention and the parent is so engrossed in their phone that they don't even notice. Very young children are now being given devices that essentially act as electronic babysitters, in addition to the modeling they see from their parents.

There are many studies, and a great deal of concern among psychologists, regarding the level of addiction present in children and young people to their devices and about the amount of time spent engaged with those devices and not in interaction with others in real time. Younger generations are losing many of their social skills and have never had the opportunity to develop others. This limits their ability to cope in real time and to solve problems, at a time when our social problems are mounting exponentially.

People have come to trust what they see on their screens more than other people or even what is happening right in front of their eyes. Given how specifically "facts," news, and information are curated for us, we are no longer living in the same world with the people next to us, and we are more than ever trapped in our own little bubbles with other people who think like we do. This limits our ability to develop empathy and divides communities that used to live by common agreement as to what constituted reality. Such division limits our understanding. We are more likely to exclude others if they don't label themselves the same as we do.

The priorities of the digitally entrained are changing as well, and I personally see this as a concern because we are losing our connection with Nature. Not only does the manufacture and disposable nature of these devices affect the environment, but the radiofrequency radiation (RF) used in the 5G technology we are moving into also affects plants and animals in a similar way to humans. It affects seedling development, the echolocation of birds, and the ability of bees, our universal pollinators, to lay eggs. I see Earth and the humans on it as all part of one big system. When we lose that connection, both humans and Earth's environment suffer and lose vibrancy. This has never been clearer than it is today, yet we seem to shove that information to the back seat in order to enjoy what technology can bring us, without even looking for a safer way to do it, unless forced to. That would cut into profits.

Certainly technology has and can be useful to our lives and our culture. But it is also changing our society in ways that are polarizing us and widening the gap between those who have and those who don't. As this book goes to print, we are in the middle of the COVID-19 crisis and have spent months engaging in remote education. Those who cannot afford technology or who are more entrained to the analog world (not a bad thing, in my mind) steadily fall behind in a world that has become more virtual. While it appears that we will move through this, back to a world that looks more familiar, remote work and schooling have gained a new foothold. It is impossible to know what the future may bring and whether there will be more global crises similar to what we are now experiencing. It has forever changed us.

As grandmothers and Wise Women, it is our role in evolution to teach the younger generations of the longer arc of time and of the rhythm beyond the day to day. The stories that we remember and tell of our earlier lives, the things we teach the young people we come into contact with, *the pace that things move when they are with us*, the attention we give them, and the value we place on real interaction all matter a great deal and can inform the younger generations. We can help to shape their brains to be able to live in the technological world without losing their ability to connect with Nature and other people.

As elder women who have gone through the process of self-evaluation and integration, we are perfectly placed to model for the young the things they are not learning in their digital world. What we know must not be lost. Consciously seeing ourselves as memory keepers can help us to focus the types of information and experience that we pass on to the young people in our lives.

Going Deeper

What Will You Give?

When you think of yourself as someone a young person would depend on to connect the past through the present to the future, is that something you move toward or away from? We bring skills and perspectives with us that are no longer possible, as our grandmothers did for us.

Our perspectives are valuable and essential right now, not just as stories of an old-fashioned time that seems quaint but as perspectives that show the need to connect with our fellow human beings in a common way, not just as polar opposites fighting over issues. Cooperation is what allows for survival and evolution, not one side prevailing over another. We need to bring the skills we were able to develop in that regard to the generations coming behind us. How can we model this? How can we convey its importance to the young ones we come in contact with? Here are some questions to consider:

- When you were young, was there a grandmother or older woman or man in your life who imparted values to you from their life and generation that were different from what you were encountering in your own life?

- What was your reaction to their perspective? Did you value it or just consider it "old-fashioned"?

- If you did not value it, is there a way it could have been shared with you that would have made you take it more seriously? How? Why?

- When you look back at your life, before technology, what do you notice has changed the most, in positive and negative ways?

- What have you lost and gained personally from the blossoming of technology?

- How have you embraced, rejected, or limited technology in your own life?

- If you have limited it, does this separate you from others around you? How does it affect your ability to relate to others?

- Go through your house and count the number of "smart" devices you own and use. Are you surprised? Do you really need them all? How does their "smartness" add to their value in your life, or would an analog version be just as useful?

- What seems worth keeping, as you add technology to your world? How and to whom do you feel it is important to transmit this knowledge?

- What are the values you would most want to transmit to the younger generations? What skills? How would you do this?

- Do the younger people you come in contact with seem to want this? How do they respond if you bring these things up?

I would encourage you to think about what values you find most important in human interaction and see as necessary to a world that allows humanity to thrive. A lot of time in this chapter focused on the virtual versus the analog world, because I see that as a fundamental shift that changes the way we relate to other humans and the Earth. We act differently when we interact virtually. It becomes easier *not* to be empathetic; to focus on our own needs and interests and create a faux community while ignoring what is happening outside our own door.

There are other things that are also disappearing. We are experiencing species extinction and destructive climate change at an alarming rate. Whole cultures are disappearing. People are being forced out of their homes and countries for political or climate reasons in numbers we have never seen and cannot integrate. The chasm between rich and poor has become so great as to beggar belief. In this country in particular, where our individual freedoms are comparatively great, if we are not in actual contact with those different from us, it becomes easy to focus only on our own needs and desires. We no longer seek out differences or opposing viewpoints but polarize, dig in our heels, and become entrenched far too easily.

Whenever your voice can be heard, give input on a project, counsel another human being, teach someone, model for them—speak your wisdom, show your heart. Bring the long arc of your knowledge to those around you. Show 'em how it's done.

Chapter 19

Begin It Now

When it comes to the future, there are three
kinds of people: those who let it happen, those
who make it happen, and those who wonder
what happened.   —John M. Richardson Jr.

I f you have done the work of this book, you should know a
lot more about yourself at this juncture. By now, you have
a pretty good idea of how you got to where you are at this
point in your life, what the influences have been that created the
current you, and how your earliest experiences continue to shape
who you are today. You also probably have a pretty good idea of
what you want to keep with you as you move forward in your life
and what you would like to add.

Insight is only a first step, though; it isn't a guarantee of change.
Just knowing why something is the way it is does not automatically mean you can shift it. That is ongoing work. Some patterns
are deeply ingrained, laid down at such an early age as to be almost
unconscious. We *can* change these, but they are often more resis-
tant than layers that have been added more recently, because of
information we have received on a subject—for instance, diet. On
the other hand, for some women, all it takes is a change in narrative to change their lives. It all ripples out from there. Doing the
self-inquiry and exercises in this book will help you to become
more aware of what your narrative is and how it was created.

Everyone is different in terms of creating a successful strategy to make the changes we want to make. Depending on our gifts, skills, and perspectives on life, some will make charts and lists; others will engage in changing microhabits or just move toward changing *what* they feel able to, *when* they feel able. Yet others will need to let this gestate for a while before doing anything and just let it settle in.

Many women put off making changes in their lives because they literally can't imagine things differently, they don't know what they want, or change seems overwhelming. It does not have to be. Actually, making changes, even small ones, simplifies life considerably. In general, we are healthiest when we live closer to the way Nature intended—real food, real activity, good sleep, human connection, and a simplified environment. What we do already is a set of habits; making change is merely creating a different set of them. Even one baby step will have a positive ripple effect on many areas of your health and well-being.

Remember, you can pull any thread and unravel the Universe. You are already on the path. Take a step, any step, and you are on your way. A vibrant life is in your hands.

You have a deeper knowledge of yourself now and a clearer picture of the possible roads ahead. As the cultural memory keepers, we remember when Nature was more balanced and vibrant with diversity. This granular connection to the physical world developed capacities in us that we are in danger of losing. We and the planet we live on are One. We are formed of the same stuff and dependent on one another for our well-being. It is important that what we know, in our minds and in our bodies, not be lost.

The Power We Hold

I think it is important to reflect on what power really is. Is it the power to kill things or take them away, or to give life and nurture it? To create fear and obedience, or to create a zone of safety where things can grow and thrive? Is it the ability to think for ourselves, without a constant barrage of influence? I don't think we realize how purposefully and powerfully we are distracted—a lot of effort and money goes into doing this. There is great value in accessing the quiet place in ourselves, deep down, where we can hear our own voice and touch base with what we know to be true. Otherwise our true voice is drowned out by the chatter.

I ask these questions because as Grandmothers who will impart the cultural memory that shapes our newest generation, we can powerfully bring our voices to this discussion. If we are whole, and know who we are, we are less easily influenced by the various agendas that vie for our attention. If we are whole, we can remember how to nurture ourselves, the people we care for, and the planet. We can bring to bear the tools we have used to understand and tell our *own* stories, to help create the story of the world to come: being present, seeing with a bold eye, relating without judgment, creating safe spaces, telling our truth, listening to others. It has never been more important for women's voices to be heard—we who work so hard to bring life into the world do not jump first to strategies that take it away.

I have always been struck by how, as humans, all of our secrets are essentially the same secret. We hold close to our chests the things we are hurt by or ashamed of, feeling that if others knew these things about us, we would be judged negatively or seen as weak or damaged. I remember being in a writing workshop where what we were writing in our exercises was to be totally unfiltered. We had to write down every single word that came into our heads and then question ourselves as to its meaning. The last step of the process was to read what we had written aloud to the group.

It was terrifying to speak aloud the unfiltered material and experiences of our lives. It was very much not what we are taught culturally. However, by the end of the weekend, I became powerfully aware that all of what we were hiding within ourselves in order to "look good" was essentially the same. We are all humans on Earth. We share a commonality of experience whether we live on opposite sides of the planet, in different cultures, or in different socioeconomic groups. We all love, hurt, desire, and have the same basic human needs. We all have the spark of the Divine in us, which wants to grow and shine and lift ourselves up, to be more, to be better. We need to begin to see that spark in others, in those who are different from ourselves. Given the level of stress in our world, we are mostly functioning out of our primitive brains, concerned with survival and "power over." We are losing the ability to have empathy for others, and we must not.

You can use this book as a tool for finding your voice, and I hope you will. I encourage you to create safe space to know others, hold one another as you explore. Meet with other women, like-minded or not, talk to one another, show yourselves to one another, do the work of becoming whole together. Let your voices be heard, whether in the circle of your family or in the wider world. It has never been more important that we bring the power of nurturing to the world where killing and taking away have come to represent power and have held sway for so long.

There is life to live, love to share, work to do. Begin it now.

Acknowledgments

This book is written with grateful thanks to all the women who have passed through my practice and my life over the last four decades and shared their dreams and desperation with me. I am inspired by you all—your courage, your insights, and your dreams.

Special thanks to my early readers, Susanne Warren, Susannah Appelbaum, and Susanrachel Condon; and to Teresa Robertson, for enduring friendship and decades of conversation about women, babies, and consciousness.

Grateful thanks to my editor, Haven Iverson, for believing in this book and helping me bring it to birth. And to the creative and professional teams at Sounds True. Though I have not met all of you, I have felt you holding me all along the way.

About the Author

S usan Willson, CNM, is a cross-cultural midwife. She has always seen the body as intelligent and capable, and has spent her career helping to support and empower women to trust their body and work with its natural intelligence. Her original degrees were in psychology and English from Emory University. Once she understood how much of our trajectory is influenced in the womb and at birth, she began her study of midwifery and returned to Emory for a nursing degree, followed by a master's degree at Yale University.

From the beginning, Willson has been interested in other cultures and what their birth traditions tell us about how they view being human. She has lived and worked among the Navajo, in Africa, and with Alaska Native, Mexican, and Pacific Rim cultures. She is always looking across a broad spectrum for what connects us as human beings, as well as the differences in each culture that add spice to the basic recipe.

Willson's last two decades have been spent working with women in the menopausal transition. Working deeply with women during this time of life strongly reinforced her view that menopause is both positive and purposeful and that it is forcefully shaped by our personal history and how we experience our female identity.

About Sounds True

Sounds True is a multimedia publisher whose mission is to inspire and support personal transformation and spiritual awakening. Founded in 1985 and located in Boulder, Colorado, we work with many of the leading spiritual teachers, thinkers, healers, and visionary artists of our time. We strive with every title to preserve the essential "living wisdom" of the author or artist. It is our goal to create products that not only provide information to a reader or listener but also embody the quality of a wisdom transmission.

For those seeking genuine transformation, Sounds True is your trusted partner. At SoundsTrue.com you will find a wealth of free resources to support your journey, including exclusive weekly audio interviews, free downloads, interactive learning tools, and other special savings on all our titles.

To learn more, please visit SoundsTrue.com/freegifts or call us toll-free at 800.333.9185.

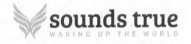

sounds true
WAKING UP THE WORLD